PRAISE FOR *DEAD RECKONING*

"Yuck! Gross! But, especially, gee whiz! Michael Baden can make dead bodies say more than talk-show guests. *Dead Reckoning* is a completely fascinating study of modern pathology, and Baden-on-autopsies never fails to astonish, educate, and (I swear) entertain."

—Jeffrey Toobin, author of *Too Close to Call*

"Candid as a Y-incision. *Dead Reckoning* describes forensic science in vivid, living color."

—Kathy Reichs, author of *Grave Secrets*

"Delightfully creepy material. . . . Baden is a methodical and ethical medical examiner and consummate scientist. . . . The account is replete with a cast of weird, amiable characters, historical insights, and reverence for the scientific study of the dead. Baden and Roach invite the outsider into the laboratory with a gripping sense of imme-diacy, and conversely, they bring the usually hidden forensic sciences into the light of day."

—*Publishers Weekly*

"This book is about the work of one of our era's foremost forensic pathologists. It is a fascinating window into the world of the medical detective."

—Tracy Kidder, author of *Home Town*

"Marion Roach and Michael Baden have written a genuinely fascinat-ing and entertaining book of tales that reveal just how garrulous the dead really are. This is the most fun you'll ever have in the morgue."

—William Kennedy

"This engaging account of former New York City medical examiner Michael Baden's intimate dealings with the dead over the past two and a half decades is full of surprises. . . . Baden and Roach deserve high praise."

—Chris Borris, *Wired*

"Drawing on cases that are famous or merely instructive, Baden imparts both the mechanics of what happens when the scalpel comes out and the paramount importance of upholding scientific objectivity during the examination. . . . True-crime buffs will be riveted by Baden's offbeat tour."

—*Booklist*

"This book is more than the cases Baden handled; it is an in-depth, engrossing look, even for the squeamish, at how medical examiners work and why you want a competent one on your side."

—*Library Journal*

Dead Reckoning

The New Science of Catching Killers

**Michael Baden, M.D.,
and Marion Roach**

A TOUCHSTONE BOOK
PUBLISHED BY SIMON & SCHUSTER
NEW YORK LONDON TORONTO SYDNEY SINGAPORE

TOUCHSTONE
Rockefeller Center
1230 Avenue of the Americas
New York, NY 10020

For information about special discounts for bulk purchases,
please contact Simon & Schuster Special Sales:
1-800-456-6798 or business@simonandschuster.com

Book design by Ellen R. Sasahara

Manufactured in the United States of America

10   9   8   7   6   5   4   3   2   1

The Library of Congress has cataloged the Simon & Schuster edition
as follows:

Baden, Michael M.
Dead reckoning : the new science of catching killers / Michael Baden
and Marion Roach.
p. cm.
Includes bibliographical references and index.
1. Homicide investigation. 2. Medical examiners (Law) 3. Forensic
sciences. 4. Forensic pathology. 5. Crime laboratories. 6. Crime scenes.
I. Roach, Marion. II. Title.
HV8079.H6 B27 2001
363.25'9523—dc21   2001040011
ISBN 0-684-86758-3
        0-684-85271-3 (Pbk)
Photographs 1, 4, 8–16 by Michael E. Baden
Names and identifying characteristics of some
individuals have been changed.

*To the forensic sciences, which can bring the guilty to justice
and the wrongly accused to freedom, and can provide for
the victims of crime some measure of peace*

———

M.B.: To Linda, Trissa, Lindsey, Sarah, Robert,
Laze—and especially Jud

M.R.: In memory of Susannah McCorkle

Contents

	Preface	9
One	*AUTOPSY*	11
Two	*BLOOD*	33
Three	*WITNESS*	57
Four	*INSIDE*	93
Five	*HENRY*	119
Six	*SCENES*	135
Seven	*BUGS*	155
Eight	*EXHUMATION*	177
Nine	*HEADS*	205
Ten	*JUNK*	227
Eleven	*RENO*	251
	Acknowledgments	269
	Sources	272
	Index	277

Preface

We were introduced in 1998 by the editor of the Albany, New York, *Times Union,* and at that first dinner we began a conversation that we have been having ever since. Marion says we get along like peanut butter and jelly. Michael likes that and agrees, although that's not the way he would say it. And there, in our difference, is the essence of our work together: We see the same things differently. Michael tends to be more contained in his descriptions; Marion never is.

Neither one of us could have written this book on his or her own. This book is most definitely the product of two sets of eyes— one in glasses, one not—looking out over the world Michael has inhabited for forty years.

What is at the core of our collaboration is a shared passion for forensic science. Marion has studied everything that Michael has grown accustomed to looking at during those forty years and then, as she says, "goes home and bleeds all over the page." Then

Michael puts it in context. Marion goes to blood school; Michael explains what it means. Marion goes to bug school; Michael interprets the importance of entomology in forensic science as well as how forensic entomology is understood in America's courts. Michael performs the autopsies and sits in the witness chair in court while Marion watches Michael in both places, notebook balanced in one palm.

At her first autopsy, Marion chose initially to sit in the only chair in the room, as far from the body as she could. But as the day went on, Michael watched her inch closer to the homicide victim and the autopsy table, watched as she got up and walked over to the process, to the story itself. And as she stood over the open body of a murdered man, Michael saw what the details of this autopsy could mean to an audience. It was right afterward that we decided to shape this book in a way that takes the reader where no reader has ever gone before: into the autopsy suite, even into the body, onto the witness stand, to blood school and bug school, and ultimately to Reno for an annual forensic science convention.

We hope you enjoy reading about these experiences as much as we enjoyed writing about them.

MICHAEL BADEN, M.D.
MARION ROACH
DECEMBER 2000

One
AUTOPSY

A good body bag gives up no clues. Little about what it contains should be detected by any of the five senses of the observer. And nothing should be presumed—not even the length of what's inside. Death, after all, changes everything. And unnatural death changes everything absolutely.

The Office of the New York City Medical Examiner orders about 8,000 body bags each year; Philadelphia's M.E., about 3,000; and Milwaukee's, about 2,000. Massachusetts offices prefer shrouds, which are more like plastic envelopes folded and welded at the ends. They order 5,000.

The same polyvinyl chloride used to make pipes can be woven into a flexible fabric of varying degrees of strength. Some body bags will be dragged over long distances of rugged underbrush; others will be hoisted on the rocker legs of helicopters. Bags may need to be nothing more than short-term storage compartments, or nothing less than unconditionally leakproof vessels of somber transport. Zippers can swoop around the edges of the bag or run right down the middle. Handles, rivets and locks are optional.

These days most body bags are white. That way you don't miss much—the red carpet fiber, the black hair, a chartreuse fleck of paint. You can see a lot, if you know how to look.

I see body bags in morgues. The morgue is usually in the basement of the hospital, far away from the elevators, the newsstand and the flower shop, but too often near the patients' kitchen. Inside the morgue is a smell that is one part tissue preservative, two parts astringent cleaner and three parts death. In the smaller morgues, against one wall there is a small, square stainless steel cooler whose door handles may or may not be locked. In larger morgues, the dead can earn a whole room. Above the door handles is a thermometer. It should read about 38 degrees Fahrenheit, above freezing but cold enough to prevent bacteria from growing and causing decomposition changes.

The autopsy suite, with its exposed pipes in the ceiling and drains in the tile floor, is lined with jars of preservative holding visible tissue and excised body parts that await their day in court. The stainless steel autopsy table is at the center of the room. A large metal grocery-type scale hangs over its foot. On the table's right side is a smaller steel table, topped with a corkboard dissecting block, the tools of the trade and some formalin-filled sample jars into which tissue will be placed.

To anyone accustomed to emergency room television shows, the utensils of the morgue are going to look big and urgent—more like hardware than surgical supply. But the concern in this room is not to bring the patient back to life; it is to speak with and for the dead. And that requires having a look and moving things around, more so than has ever been depicted on any television show. There you see scalpels. Here, lying next to the scalpels, are a bread knife, pruning clippers and a vibrating bone saw.

On any given morning in a hospital morgue, funeral directors may drop in and out: signing in, talking to me, drinking coffee, eating a donut, then signing out and taking away the bodies that have been released. The morgue can be a busy and friendly place.

Those present during a homicide autopsy will usually include the police working the crime, an assistant district attorney, the *diener* (pronounced DEE-ner, the old German title for the autopsy assistant), the body and me. Sometimes a few others might be there—a police photographer and maybe a forensic pathologist, a forensic nurse or an emergency medical student in training.

Chances are good that I will know the detectives and that we've worked together before. High-fives may be exchanged among the police over a conviction in a recent case, and memories of convictions past will be recalled. The friendliness diminishes some of the depressing aspects of the morgue. But too much friendship and you lose perspective. It's a difficult balance for the medical examiner: The prosecutors want the doctor to be part of the team; the medical examiner, though paid by the taxpayers, just as cops and prosecutors are, needs to be independent and neutral. The cops and DAs speak of the triumvirate, or the three-legged stool—lose one leg and you lose the case.

Unfortunately, many medical examiners think of themselves that way, as part of the prosecution team. It's so easy to fall into that frame of mind. The cops say, "Hey, if you can place the time of death at 3 A.M., we've got this guy cold. After that he's got an alibi." And then you start hearing about all the hideous things the "bad guy" has supposedly done in his life, while viewing all the bad things that someone did to this body on the table before you. But I have to be alert to what will guide me and what might mislead me because sometimes, of course, the cops have got it wrong.

One of the detectives will start a running monologue. I want to know what is known. And although I cannot accept what he says as certain documentation of what happened, his perspective permits me to gauge the general direction in which the autopsy should go, because the kinds of questions being raised will direct the extent to which I dissect the body. The detective tells me who the body is. Who last spoke to him. What seems to have happened. When the body was found. And where. The questions go back and forth between me and the detectives.

As the detective is talking, I will be thinking about the present as well as the future: What should I be doing now that I will be asked about in court in six months? What human tissue and fluid samples should I take? What could be misleading me here that will be obvious later once the complete circumstances of the crime are known? And, of course, what if the complete circumstances are never known, and all we will ever have is the body that is about to come out of the cooler, with its trace evidence and cause of death waiting to be discovered? I am to determine how the death occurred. At this point none of us may know why it happened.

That's the challenge every day in the morgue. And so, here we are, on this particular Tuesday morning, a few of us gathered in the basement of a New York hospital—a place similar to what is found in virtually every county of the country—to see what science may reveal about a body brought in the night before.

Getting together like this is a better system than reading police reports and making phone calls. Right now everybody who needs to be here is in the room. And those who are not here are easy to reach. The detectives are on their walkie-talkies to the police team scouring the scene where the body was found so that questions can be asked and answered. The cops tell me that the body was found faceup on the living-room carpet. I remind them to sample the carpet to determine whether or not the fibers match those on the body.

"Done it, Doc."

Maybe during the autopsy I'll want to know what's in the deceased's medicine chest or what he left in a pan on the stove. The food or drugs may or may not match what's in the stomach, and that could speak to time of death. You never can tell what you might want to know. But you always start with what you *do* know.

It seems that at some point during a recent national holiday, while many Americans were busy peeling vegetables and folding linen napkins, the man in the body bag in the cooler died in his own home. He was found several days later. Probably a homicide, too soon to tell. His car was stolen and sold, maybe by the perpetrator, maybe not. It was later recovered. This much is known. And then the conversation dies away.

Everything becomes quiet when the lock comes off the cooler.

One of the detectives writes the time on a legal pad as the diener wheels the transport gurney over and slides out the bag. The diener then pushes the gurney over to the autopsy table and shifts the body bag onto it. In German, the word *diener* has many meanings, including "attendant," "responsible manservant" and "slave." In the course of a day, an American diener will cut, saw, clean and sew. First, he unzips the bag.

If there are any fainters, this is when they go. There's a rule of thumb: The bigger the cop, the faster they drop. It's the smell. District attorneys don't go down much. But they tend to hold on to the wall and the backs of chairs and hang back behind the others. The exception is women, who usually do just fine.

The autopsy table has two tiers. The top, on which the corpse lies, is a metal sheet, perforated to allow flowing water and body fluids to seep through to the bottom level, which is also metal and serves as a catch basin. Running water is an essential element in an autopsy room. It flows over the bottom tier of the table, continually rinsing it clean. This is a great improvement over one table I worked on in New York City's Bellevue Hospital forty years ago. It was made of three-inch-thick solid marble and had absorbed decades of body fluids.

My mind has to be very clear now. If it isn't, I have to clear it consciously. No more thinking about the kids, the move, the bills, the news, the next autopsy, the last autopsy, but only about this autopsy, right here—this body, which, in itself, is a crime scene.

This mental clearing begins with suiting up in the locker room. Autopsy attire consists of the green or blue extra-large scrub suits discarded by the surgeons on the upper floors of the hospital. Washed and sterilized, of course, but secondhand all the same, they are sent down to the basement, just like the dead. To have more room to maneuver, it is best to wear big scrubs. There is a lot more comfort when the scrubs are big. This is physical work, and it's a long day. Autopsies require removing clothing, cutting, sawing, lifting, dissecting, weighing, examining and turning over bodies, all done while standing, sometimes for as long as twelve hours. So it's good to be comfortable in the well-worn scrubs, under the disposable plastic apron. The thin, extra-large latex gloves are teased out of the cardboard box, and I snap them on. The booties I slip over my shoes. And by then, my mind should be clear.

Down goes the body bag zipper. Up go the masks on some of the people in the room. Those who wear them use the stiff, white masks—the kind you use when you sand furniture, the ones with the metal band across the nose to crimp. Those who don't want the smell in their noses pass around a small bottle of wintergreen oil and rub some on the inside of the masks to cut the odor. (They won't realize until later that the smell of death and decomposition will be carried home with them anyway, on their clothes and in their hair.) The wintergreen oil will be passed around a lot this morning; the smell of this man indicates that he's been dead for a while.

Smell is important in an autopsy. Many of the younger medical examiners wear rebreather devices because the Federal Occupational Safety and Health Administration (OSHA) says they have to. And because of that, they miss a lot. The bitter almond odor of cyanide, for instance, retells the tale of a poisoning.

Only about 50 percent of the population can smell cyanide. The ability to do so is genetic, like rolling your tongue. It's a good quality for a medical examiner to have, especially around

Halloween, in case someone has been lacing candy with cyanide, or as during the Tylenol scare, when certain bottles were contaminated and a good nose would have identified which ones. But no one can smell cyanide, or much of anything else, while wearing a rebreather.

Alcohol can also be smelled at autopsy. All alcohol—from Sneaky Pete to Dom Perignon, it makes no difference—is ethanol. Regardless of its original form, ethanol has a uniquely distinct sweet smell. It's another of the body's great equalizers, reducing rotgut as well as the smoothest single malt to its lowest common denominator. Smell alone can't determine the amount someone drank, but it can say if alcohol was present at the time of death, as is the case in about 40 percent of unnatural deaths: drunk driving, accidental falls, fires, suicides, drownings, homicides, fights at home, bar brawls. It's there a lot, and you can smell it in the dead.

There was a time when people drank gasoline to kill themselves, and it was easy to smell. But then in the 1950s barbiturates came along, and people looking to die switched over to pills. The suicide rate didn't fall. People always seem to find ways to die.

The fact is that we die as we live. This is especially true when death is due to unnatural causes. The body reflects the good and harmful things done to it over a lifetime—cigarettes smoked, alcohol drunk, glasses worn (even contacts change the shape of the eye), drugs taken, preferences in sexual activity, stress, exercise and chosen method of suicide. The range of human appetites and desires can be seen in, on and under the skin. All of this can be read at death like a biography.

The man inside the bag on the autopsy table died maybe as long ago as a week, maybe less if he was left near a heater. After death, the body changes in ways that help us determine the time of death. The changes post death are rigor mortis, algor mortis and livor mortis, but they are not precise. Because the heart is no longer pumping, muscle cells are deprived of oxygen and they stiffen. This is called rigor mortis. The body temperature falls one to two degrees Fahrenheit per hour. This is called algor mortis. And because the heart is no longer churning the blood, the red blood cells settle according to gravity and produce the maroon color of death on the skin, or livor mortis. Rigor mortis begins at the lower jaw and neck and spreads downward. The first medical person to the scene will usually feel the jaw and note the rigidity. The whole body will be stiff within twelve hours after death. Thirty-six hours after death, the stiffening will have disappeared. Heat, cold and drugs can affect the way the body changes after death. Heat speeds things up. A detective confirms that the heat was on pretty high in the apartment where this man was found.

The body was wrapped in a white hospital sheet that was brought to the crime scene by the detectives. You shouldn't wrap a body in sheets from the victim's house. Doing so could transfer material from another part of the residence into the crime scene and would confuse things. With a clean sheet brought to the scene, anything that falls on it will have come from the victim and perhaps whomever he came in contact with during those last moments of his life.

Before the decedent is removed from the body bag, a search must be made of the bag. It might reveal something—the bullet that had shaken loose of a wound of Governor John Connally after going through President John F. Kennedy and was found on a stretcher, for instance—or it might show nothing. If the body was wrapped properly, there should be little information in the bag— it should be inside the sheet and on the body. But you always check.

We then lift the stiff legs and inch the bag down the table, sliding it out from under the body inside the white sheet. As the sheet is unwrapped, I see a black man, approximately 5 feet 10 inches tall, weighing about 140 pounds. There are balloonlike brown paper bags around the hands and feet. Tied at the wrists and ankles, they entrap any trace evidence that might be on the hands and feet. Virtually anything could be a clue—fibers, bullets, chewing gum on a shirt, a cigarette butt on the heel of a shoe, flecks of paint, garden soil or sand beneath a fingernail.

Criminalistics is the scientific examination of physical evidence for legal purposes. It is one of the forensic sciences. Others include the obvious specialties, such as psychiatry, dentistry, fingerprint analysis and toxicology, as well as the not so obvious: engineering, entomology, botany, geology and climatology. All can be used to prove an argument in court.

And that is the ultimate point of all of the forensic sciences in criminal cases: To find anything that will incriminate or exclude a suspect and then to argue successfully in court that with these traces of evidence it can be proved to a reasonable degree of scientific certainty that a specific crime was or was not committed by a specific person. The trace evidence may be the difference between sending someone away for life or sending someone home. And it may be minuscule.

When you walk into a room, you change it. In fact, how you enter and exit changes things. Enter, turn around and walk right out, touching nothing, and you have still left something of yourself behind—a grain of sand from the sole of your shoe, perhaps, or a fiber from the carpet of your car. It could be a hair—yours or that of someone you touched earlier.

Enter a room and have a physical fight with someone, and you will change that room, yourself and the other person by what you exchange. It's very simple: When any two objects come into contact with each other, there is always a transfer from one object to the other. This is called Locard's Exchange Principle, and it is the basis of the science of criminalistics: what was left behind, what was taken away, what was exchanged. Find it and you may solve the crime.

But before you open the bags on the hands and feet or even make a complete sweep of the sheet, you've got to check the tag.

In every death there will be at least one tag somewhere on the body, usually on a toe, a wrist or an ankle—if those limbs exist.

People think in terms of toe tags, but they also tend to think in terms of clean, naked bodies, or at least naked feet, which is not always the case. The idea is to place the tag where it is least likely to disturb anything. In today's case it is on the left ankle above the bag.

The first tag will be placed on the body by the person who is going to move that body from the scene. A second tag will be put on in the receiving morgue. That way a chain of evidence—and a record of who has touched the body—is begun.

People who die in hospitals will also have wrist tags. Usually, however, nurses will remove any intravenous lines and tubes after a death. Medical examiners would prefer that the body appear in the morgue as it had at the time of death, tubes and all, in case there is any question of whether or not they were inserted properly. But nurses and hospital managers are concerned with neatness, not evidence. The same thing happens all the time in the emergency room when clothes from a crime scene are cut away and discarded, even on live victims. We need the clothes. We need anything that might tell the tale of the crime.

Bodies coming down from hospital floors are wrapped in white plastic or white sheets, both to prevent contamination and to shield onlookers from the sight. The wrapped body comes into the refrigerated part of the morgue, awaiting instructions from the family to the funeral director. When the funeral director comes in, all he sees is the toe tag.

Bodies do get mixed up. A car crash can leave one person dead and another up on a hospital ward in a coma, fully bandaged, and it may not be until the person in the coma awakes that someone realizes the person buried in the ground was misidentified. Only small-town funeral directors know their clients and even then mistakes are made, especially with babies, who are very hard to tell apart.

That was the case with two babies in upstate New York who remain buried under the wrong names to this day. One was murdered. The other just happened to die of natural causes in the hospital on the same day. It was not until years later, when the grave of the murdered child was opened and the body exhumed, that the mistake was discovered. We knew immediately because the child was the wrong sex. The DA at the time decided it would prove more hardship than not to tell the other set of parents. He ordered the child quietly reburied in the wrong grave.

The wrong bodies also end up in graves when families come in to identify their loved ones but can't bear to open their eyes for the actual viewing. Since the police have just informed the family members that a loved one is dead, they take that to be true and sometimes just seem to peer through their hands, shaking their heads, while they are actually not looking. A few days later at the funeral home viewing they may be terribly surprised to discover that the dead person is not their family member at all. It has happened.

Other confusion can arise if the person is not dead. The freshly dead human body looks much like a person who is asleep. Once in a while, however, a live one wakes up in the morgue. It happened at Albany Medical Center in upstate New York not long ago, when a man awakened and shouted, "What am I doing here?"— and nearly scared the diener to death. That being the case, right after I check the toe tag, I listen for a heartbeat.

Then, if there is a wallet, I check the driver's license photo and hold it next to the face.

In the driver's license photo of the body on the table on this day, the dead man is smiling. But now his dark skin is turning green. A detective talks about him. Only a week before, the man was volunteering his time, befriending the needy, buying a new car and planning a holiday dinner with his family.

Now he is lying atop a white sheet, on a perforated stainless steel slab, fully clothed in the muted hues of the season. The neck of his shirt is unbuttoned, and it exposes at least one point of transfer from the perpetrator to the victim. Around the man's neck is an alarm clock cord entwined with a dehumidifier cord, both with their two-prong plugs intact.

Along with a photograph, the driver's license can provide the height of the deceased. But many people lie about their height, especially those who are short. And relatives frequently are mistaken about one another's height. We measure height carefully in the morgue. Getting it wrong can cause real problems.

When Lee Harvey Oswald was autopsied, his height and weight were recorded along with the other findings of the medical examiner. After Oswald was buried, a British author published a book in which he claimed that a Russian imposter was actually buried in Oswald's grave. He based his assertion on several facts: The height of the body in the grave differed from that recorded on Oswald's license, and likewise, Oswald had a mastoid scar behind his right ear that had gone unnoticed or unrecorded in the autopsy report. Before penicillin, removing a portion of the mastoid bone behind the ear was a necessary treatment for mastoiditis—a bacterial infection, then common in children. Apparently, this was the case with Oswald when he was a child. The body was eventually re-autopsied, and dental records confirmed that it was, indeed, that of Lee Harvey Oswald. But the entire unnecessary ordeal only fanned the flames of the John F. Kennedy assassination controversy.

So you want to get it right the first time.

Following the measured height and estimated weight, photographs are taken from every angle. In this case that includes numerous close-ups of the ligature, which is not tight. In fact, it's almost draped around the neck of the man. If he had been conscious, he could have removed it. After looking at and feeling the cords, looking under them for abrasions, noting their positions on the neck, I remove them and place them in an evidence bag. The time is noted.

A detective says the man is gay. His medical records reveal that he is HIV-positive. The fact that the ligature is not tight, the cops are saying, could speak to rough sex that went bad. I tune them out, putting aside anything that might misdirect my thinking. The police want it to be a clear case of homicide that no defense attorney can undermine. Of course they do. It's their job. But that might not be what happened.

Yes, it could have been rough sex. It could have been consensual rough sex. It could have been that the ligature was slipped on after death to lead any investigation astray. It could be many things, especially when sex is concerned.

There are incalculable ways people get into trouble with sex and end up in the hospital, both dead and alive. I start telling the cops about that couple all those years ago in Manhattan who weren't married to each other (but were married to other people) who came into the ER at Bellevue that night. He was carrying her wrapped around the front of him, facing him. They were both naked, with a coat thrown over her.

The cops aren't listening carefully. They are opening brown paper evidence bags and standing them open on the floor, in lines, ready to take in evidence. Nobody has looked over. After all, it's just another tale told over a dead man. Everyone in the room has heard a million of them, it seems.

Must have been some cab ride over to Bellevue, I say. Then there's that long walk to the hospital off the avenue. Her legs were wrapped right around his hips. Turns out they had been having sex.

The cops finally look interested.

They were stuck. Her IUD was hooked into his foreskin.

The cops wince.

In the case on the table today, there is a recent medical file entry for an emergency room visit when the man's tongue got caught in his dentures.

"Oral sex," says one of the cops, like he's laying down a bet.

Everything that happened at the scene is reviewed. The cops say, for instance, that they cut the appliances away from the end of the cords but did nothing else to disrupt the evidence, except, of course, transport the body here to the morgue. They wrapped the body in a hospital sheet, then in the body bag, and brought it here.

Looks like the cops did a good job. Not like the O.J. Simpson case, where the LAPD detectives stepped in the blood of the murder victims, tracking it all over the place. You can see it in the crime photos. What a disaster. This one is all by the book, nicely done, as it should be.

This autopsy began at 11:15 A.M. At 12:24 P.M., the bags come off the hands. Each bag goes into an evidence bag marked RIGHT or LEFT. Fingernail scrapings are taken. If there was a struggle, there might be hair or skin under the nails. The veins in the hands are bulging, as they do in the recently dead. They do this in the living, as well, whenever the hands are lower than the rest of the body. Whenever I see this, I always think of how beautifully Rembrandt captured this in his anatomical drawings.

But the hands here are beginning to wither. Fingerprinting may be tough going as a result, but that's not done until all the specimens are collected.

Then it's time to turn out the overhead lights. I use what is called a Woods Light to search the clothes and body for semen, which fluoresces under ultraviolet rays. Blood and saliva will not fluoresce. Some lint does, though. As I direct the Woods Light, which is the size of a large flashlight, over the body, odd patterns and splotches of purplish white light appear.

At 12:31 P.M., lunch is wheeled in.

The lights go back on.

"Hey, Doc, want a sandwich?" Ham sandwiches, caffeinated sodas. Hospital fare on a stainless steel cart. This might be the absolute extreme fringe of machismo, eating ham sandwiches in a morgue. Maybe not, but it is a good time for the cops to take a break and a good time for me to think out loud into my handheld tape recorder, while things are still fresh. These notes will become the autopsy report, transcribed and typed and distributed for trial.

Look and see, talk and record, walk around and around the

body, touching only what is necessary, having a look, poking the skin on the bloated face to see if there is slippage, or the separation of the outer layer of skin from the inner layers. There is some, meaning he's at medium decomposition. The skin seems almost ready to tear. Holding the dead man's hand, looking at the hands, getting it down on tape in precise detail so no one can question what was there and what wasn't. All of this is important.

Jewelry will be noted: what it is and where it is worn. Making no assumptions about value, everything gets reduced on record to "yellow metal," "white metal," "a white stone in a gray metal setting." Shoe color, the presence of socks, open or closed cuffs, clothing label and sizes, all are recorded right here with the color and position of the ligature, the green color of the sagging skin and the protruding, drying tongue of the deceased. It all goes on the record.

Collecting samples from this body requires a rape kit, which contains tubes for fluid collection, envelopes for scrapings and hair, and swabs with corresponding containers to protect them from contamination. After a swab is used, it is suspended in a cardboard box that holds it firmly so that nothing touches the tip. Tiny envelopes hold individual hairs, fingernails, fibers. Vials hold blood or urine.

While DNA must be preserved dry to avoid deterioration, swabs may have to be wet in order to pick up such evidence. Then they have to be dried, preserved and analyzed. A lot of medical examiners insist on using distilled water to moisten swabs. They don't want any contamination of foreign substances. I think it's a little silly. Tap water is fine. There's lots of stuff in city water, but sperm isn't one of them. And right now we're swabbing for sperm.

The next thing to do is turn off the air conditioner so that no little fibers or hairs get blown away. The room is instantly hot, still and smelly. The smell is so dense that it seems you can feel it in the air. The little bottle of wintergreen oil is passed around again.

"That stuff stinks," says the diener, nodding toward the oil. He is not wearing a mask.

After lunch the exacting process of picking fiber evidence off the dead man will begin. Trace evidence collection is slow going. One hair at a time goes into little envelopes, which are marked and timed. A few hairs are plucked from the scalp as well as from the graying mustache. They come out easily at this stage of decomposition, with barely a tug. Everything goes into the rape kit.

The door to the morgue swings open, and two people breeze in carrying candy-apple red blankets. They are here to pick up a very large body, which has been lying in wait under a sheet in the small entry room between the autopsy suite and the locker and shower room.

"Hiya, Doc!" says the woman, waving her arm with a blanket in its crook, the name of a local funeral parlor signaling back and forth like a pennant in the airless room. After checking the toe tag (but not looking at the body), they tighten the straps and attachments securing the blankets over the corpse and go back the way they came.

The cell phone holder worn on the belt of the dead man on the table is removed and preserved once it has been noted for the record. His pockets are checked. Inside the left front pocket of his trousers is a pillbox containing several Viagras and a couple of Wellbutrins.

The cops want to know about strangulation and erections. It's a common misconception that you always get an erection in a strangulation.

"That's bullshit, right Doc?" asks one detective through a yawn as he marks the time on the pad. A cop picks up the camera and takes pictures. Each one is marked on the pad with its time. I also take pictures, although we may emphasize different aspects of the body.

Photography was one of the first forensic sciences: Documenting crime scenes is as old as photography. In fact, the only record we have of some crimes are the photos. Evidence of the Jack the Ripper murder scenes of 1888, for instance, exists today only on film. Photography remains an essential tool in the morgue as well as at the crime scene.

The clothes are wrestled off the corpse and each article placed in a bag with the time marked. There is chewing gum, stuck to the back of the shirt, right between where the shoulder blades would be. It's a big wad, the color of what we used to call British racing green. It might be from the perpetrator, and if it is, it's going to contain his DNA. It also might retain his teeth marks. Saliva is the best source of DNA. The gum goes in the rape kit. The time is noted on the pad.

The cops radio their pals at the crime scene again and have them check to see if the man was a gum chewer, if there is any unchewed gum around anywhere. Also they should check on that carpet sample they recovered from under the body. In fact, the cops on the other end of the radio are reminded to double-check that it *was* the carpet directly under the body that was collected and brought out for evidence.

These are good cops. They know what they're doing. The landlord is going to be annoyed because of the hole in the carpet, but these guys know how to work a scene.

Shoes, socks, pants, underwear, all come off. And there it is, the naked body of a man, bloated and mottled with death, the bruises from his last encounter with another human ringing his neck.

A black rubber block is placed under the upper back, raising the throat and tilting back the head. Arching back the head makes the dead man's blackened, dried tongue slightly protrude. If this were a painting, it would be Gothic and would probably hang in the basement of a church.

We call the hospital imaging department for a portable X-ray machine, and soon a perky female X-ray technician wheels it in. Everybody knows her. She's a cop's wife, and she doesn't even blanch at the sight of the decomposing naked man stretched before her, awaiting her attention.

She takes head, neck and chest X rays, and in minutes has them developed and ready to be reviewed, along with a second set for the police to hold for potential use at trial.

The cops yawn some more, drink sodas and mark time.

The swabs come out.

"Swab of head of penis," says one cop, as I affix the specimen inside the rape kit box. Another cop marks the time as, in his best Julia Child falsetto, he repeats, "'Swab of head of penis.' Sounds like something you get in a restaurant in New York," followed by three simultaneous failed attempts to stifle laughter. Morgue humor is as much a part of the autopsy room as the head saw. And as necessary.

The lights go off again and out comes the Woods Light.

"He's glowing."

"See?" says one of the detectives. "Break your neck, you ejaculate. Told ya."

Not all comments require a response. In fact, it's possible that the sperm is left over from sex and that the perpetrator zipped up the dead man's trousers. If I am asked while on the witness stand if it is possible that there is a pink elephant in the lobby, I will reply that it is, in fact, possible. Anything is possible, and to think otherwise closes the mind to the range of human behavior. And you should never do that, especially in crimes involving sex. The mind is the largest sex organ, and anything that pops into it may—and, in my experience, can—be enacted. After all, there is nothing like orgasm for positive reinforcement of an idea.

The white sheet is removed from under the body. The body is washed.

If there are wounds, this is when they will be examined, measured for length and width, and photographed, first against a standard, 18 percent gray forensic ruler that permits accurate color development, and then without it. But there are no external wounds here.

This is also a good time to look for tattoos. Any cop will tell you that the history of a person can be read by his tats.

Tats, or tacs, or ink, the cops call them. Reading ink is a valuable recognition and interpretation skill for the medical examiner. In the case of an unknown body it can unlock the identity: Some armed forces tattoos may even include name, rank and serial number. A convict's tattoo, or joint tat, can be just as revealing and can tell me who he is, where he's been and what he's done.

Some joint tattoos are applied to hide needle marks. Others brag of a long life of drug use and will include a detailed design of a needle and syringe. Joint tats are of two types: freehand and homemade machine. The medium can be ink from a pen or cigarette ash, and it is injected under the skin point by point, in little dots, to form a picture or a word.

Homemade machines may consist of a small motor, a hollowed-out ballpoint pen, guitar string and some India ink. They allow for more detail of design. And that's where the information is.

For instance, a clock face without hands means doing time, as do spider webs on elbows or shoulders. A happy face twinned with a crying face means play now, pay later. A man emblazoned with the face of a crying female means there is someone waiting on the outside. The Mexican Mafia, Aryan brotherhood, black guerrillas, Southerners, Northerners, all manners of groups have distinguishing inks.

Words and phrases can be spelled out on knuckles, but it helps to know how to spell. I once saw F.U.K.C. across four knuckles, which appeared to be a typo, since the *K* and *C* were crossed out and re-tattooed on the opposite fingers. Several times I've seen BORN TO LOSE changed to BORN TO LOVE and men's backs covered with elaborate scenes. A huge Madonna de Guadalupe is popular across the backs of Hispanic men as a turnoff to sodomizers. The flip side of this was a tattoo I saw at autopsy of a hunt scene, complete with a fox escaping between the deceased's buttocks.

Other tattoos tell other tales. There was the man not long ago who had YOUR NAME tattooed on his penis. When I asked his brother about it, he said that the deceased was an alcoholic who had fallen on bad times. (The internal exam showing severe cirrhosis of the liver confirmed this.) Apparently the man would bet strangers at the bar the price of a drink: "I have your name tattooed on my penis." That's how he supported the drinking habit that finally killed him.

Lividity of the skin can be mistaken for tattoos, for bruises and, in the O.J. Simpson case, for a shoe print. Also known as livor mortis, lividity is the dark red, almost purplish discoloration that is seen in the skin where the blood has pooled. It is caused by the settling of the blood into the lowest parts of the body (hanging victims will have fixed lividity in their legs, for instance) and will reflect whatever the body was resting on at the time of death: rocks, the swirling patterns of bedsheets, clothing.

Lividity appears about two hours after death, so it can speak to time of death as well as reveal whether a body was moved after the person died. In that case, a corpse might, for instance, be found on its back with fixed lividity on its front. This would mean that someone turned the body over several hours after death. Lividity appears in hues of red: Cherry pink is the color of carbon monoxide poisoning, for instance. Maroon is normal.

With Wayne, the diener, assisting, we roll today's body onto its side and do a full examination of the back. Then the body will be turned again to lie naked, clean and faceup atop the perforated stainless steel table, the arms at rest by its side. The head will be centered on the black rubber block. A glance around the room and it looks like everyone is ready.

And then the scalpel is raised.

Two

BLOOD

Walking the broad, tree-lined streets of Corning, New York, at twilight in early May may be one of the great hidden delights of the world. Just when the forsythia has passed from yellow to green and the lilacs are engorged with buds, the gracious homes on the hill overlooking the Chemung River fling open their doors to the evening air. Sounds from inside the large houses mingle with spring birdsong. After an upstate winter, it is good to hear the hum of lives being lived.

Walking along the residential side streets, you pass the congressman's house, where a tennis ball can be heard hitting a clay court behind a high hedge. Over there in the perennials limning the home of the director of the Rockwell Museum is a breathtaking selection of garden glass. On a street below is the sturdy house in which Pyrex was first tested. You can almost imagine this last scene: A kitchen filled with odds and ends of glassware. A researcher from Corning comes home bearing yet another piece at which his wife looks askance. "Try it," he urges as he hands it to her, promising that, really, this version can stand up to her meat loaf.

It's easy to imagine because so many stories told in this town include Corning International Corporation, the company that makes this place what it is and which sets the tone for so much of what goes on. Corning International's Glass Museum claims to be the third most popular tourist site in the state of New York, but despite its very magnificence, it is almost rivaled by the immaculately beautiful corporate headquarters itself, shimmering under its darkly rippled high-gloss roof, on the banks of the Chemung. The company's wealth and power transfuse the town with a splendid grace and an almost opulent culture. And Corning's motto— "Discovering Beyond Imagination"—extends far outside the corporation's shiny halls. For as many in this town know well, there are events in Corning that do, in fact, extend beyond the imagination of most people.

Toward downtown, the hill of homes reaches ground level as the signs of commerce appear: shops, a hotel, a parking lot filled with cars. Near the Radisson Hotel, some people can be seen putting little red-and-white tickets on their dashboards. On closer inspection, the pattern on the cards looks like splattered polka dots, or spin-art paintings done in a monochromatic red hue. But on even closer examination, that red becomes very, very red— blood red, in fact. And there's a good reason for that: Inside the Union Hall, Herb MacDonell is busy making and distributing the parking passes by drizzling human blood onto little white cards.

Blood school, it seems, is in spring session.

The thirty or so cars marked with these parking passes are in no danger of being ticketed or towed. These are the cars of law enforcement professionals who have come from around the world to attend the weeklong basic training session at the Institute on the Physical Significance of Human Bloodstain Evidence, taught twice a year by the institute's director, Herbert Leon MacDonell, and his assistant, Paul Erwin Kish. They also offer an advanced course, Geometric Interpretation of Bloodstain Pattern Analysis, but for this first week of May, the primer course is on the agenda.

Inside the discreet walls of the Union Hall, Herb MacDonell is holding forth. He is in his element in front of the room: One minute he's modeling a shirt soaked and dried in blood, explaining to the group precisely how the blood of a murdered man sprayed up inside the cuffs; a little later he's wielding a hatchet, casting off drops of blood in the directions of his thrust and backswing. As he walks back and forth in front of his current class, he is talking, always talking, telling the class what it needs to know about the way blood drips, drops, falls, spatters, cascades, dries, shoots and travels on a flat surface, and about its velocity as it pumps out of the heart and sprays out of a severed artery and lands on every surface known to man and woman.

He is a walking, talking text on blood, and he will be the first to tell you that nobody does it better. In fact, he visibly bristles at being referred to as the country's leading authority on bloodstain. He is the *world's* leading authority on blood pattern analysis, as he has stated for the record hundreds of times on the witness stand. And it doesn't require actually reading his thirteen-page résumé —although it's a good read—to learn that he has testified in such high-profile cases as the assassinations of Robert F. Kennedy and Dr. Martin Luther King, Jr., the Black Panther case of 1969, Jean Harris's killing of the Scarsdale Diet doctor, and the O.J. Simpson case, and has been consulted in cases including the Oklahoma City bombing, the Sam Sheppard murder case, the Jeffrey MacDonald murder case, the Wayne Williams multiple murders in Atlanta, the charges against Claus von Bulow and the killing of Amadou Diallo by four New York City police officers. Because he'll be the first to tell you all about them and practically anything and everything else that comes into his mind. Herb is one hell of a talker.

Which is good, because Herb MacDonell has been called upon in his professional career to testify in thirty-four states and five foreign countries, including, as he likes to say, Los Angeles. The disciplines in which he has given expert testimony include: fingerprint identification, firearms identification, crime scene reconstruction, Breathalyzer operation (he was the first expert witness to get the Breathalyzer introduced into a New York State court), clinical symptoms of alcohol impairment, footwear identification, light microscopy, scanning electron microscopy, forensic photography, hair and fiber identification, glass and glass fracture and analytical chemistry. And he can do so because while he describes himself as a physical scientist, he has worked and studied all his life across the scientific spectrum.

His lifelong fascination with fingerprints, for instance, began when he got his first fingerprint kit at age seven. Some thirty years later he would patent the MAGNA™ Brush and accompanying magnetic fingerprinting powder that are recognized as one of the more important developments in criminalistics. Prior to that, the process of dusting for prints—with its harsh direct application of powder to brush and brush to prints—often destroyed delicate latent (or unseen) fingerprints. Herb's invention combined his knowledge of glass, lampworking, chemistry, magnetism and criminalistics, producing a fingerprint kit that is now a household tool in the world of solving crime.

But most people know him for blood and his expert testimony on bloodstain pattern analysis. In fact, he says he was the first to introduce bloodstain evidence into the courts of twenty-three states and into Canada as well as Germany. And so when the topic is blood, his name will come up, and when it does, conversation quickly turns to the school, because word is that his blood school is quite a show, led by a consummate showman.

Sitting in the morning lecture, a first-time visitor to blood school might have trouble listening to Herb MacDonell. The room is distracting, after all, with fourteen large experiment stations hemming in the listeners: to the left, a set of tables laid end to end, covered in blood-spattered paper; behind that, a huge box constructed of connected PVC pipe that has been surrounded on four sides—the floor, two of the four walls and all of the ceiling—in brown paper, running off a large roll onto the floor, a blood-stained hatchet hung casually over one of the pipes; a table on which there has been tossed a confounding collection of wigs, mismatched shoes and sneakers, whisk brooms, knives and a newel post; on another table, a stationary rifle set up to fire into a bullet trap, the box of which is itself layered inside with the explosive patterns of blood; concrete and tile samples scattered on the floor in one section; and at the front of the room, a large carton labeled RUSH: HUMAN BLOOD waiting unopened.

The idea here is to learn to interpret bloodstain evidence through the examination of the size, shape and distribution of bloodstains. This school is not about genetic markers such as DNA and ABO blood typing. This school is about reading the crime scene based on the blood that was left behind and reconstructing the events as the bleeding occurred and afterward.

Most people usually say that blood was shed or spilled. The reality of a crime scene is that while it may be sprayed, spattered, dropped, transferred, projected, cast off or gushed from one person and may soak onto another, it is neither shed nor spilled from the human body. Blood loss is more active than that. And that is due to the heart.

The heart is a pump, about the size of your fist. It is a four-chambered muscle that circulates blood. Oxygen-depleted blood returns from the body's veins into the upper chamber on the right side, or atrium, and drops into the lower chamber, or right ventricle, where it is pumped through the pulmonary artery and into the lungs. In the lungs, blood gives off the waste product carbon dioxide and takes in new oxygen. It moves on through the pulmonary veins, enters the upper chamber on the left side of the heart, the left atrium, and then drops into the lower chamber, or left ventricle, and is pumped back out into the body through the aorta, the body's largest artery.

Circulation in the human body is a nutrient delivery and waste management system. Blood brings nutrition and carries away waste. All the trillions of cells in the body need nutrients, and all of them produce waste that must be carried away. The five to six quarts of blood in each human body do this beautifully.

Approximately 55 percent of the blood in a body is plasma, a saltwater liquid. The other 45 percent is blood cells—red, white and platelets. The red cells transport oxygen from the lungs throughout the body; white cells are the body's immune defense system; and platelets help the blood to clot. During life, the beating heart not only pumps blood to every cell of the body but also churns the components so that blood cells and plasma are uniformly mixed. When the heart—the pump—stops, the mixing process stops as well, and the blood settles, which is what causes lividity, the postmortem maroon discoloration of the body.

Prick your finger and a drop of blood will rise out from the skin. Turn your finger facedown and eventually the blood will fall with gravity. Shake your hand and it will be cast off in the direction of the energy behind it. Touch something and the blood will be transferred from you to what you touch. When blood leaves the body and lands on a carpet, a shirt, an air conditioner, a floor tile, the ceiling, a bathroom floor, under someone's nails, in the cuffs of his trousers, on the backseat of a car, on a windshield or anyplace else, its behavior will follow the laws of physical science, specifically that of ballistics, or the study of projectiles in motion.

Consider again that drop of blood hovering under your downturned finger, ready to fall. Like all liquids, it is held together by forces that produce a surface resistant to penetration or separation. In fact, a drop of blood will not break up unless it is acted upon by another force, breaking its surface tension. The surface tension greatly affects the dynamics of blood by producing a force across the liquid that decreases its surface area. It actually tightens it and holds it there, like a little dome.

For a drop of blood to fall it must be large enough that its weight overcomes its surface tension. As it falls, it will oscillate and assume a spherical shape. Artists get it wrong: Raindrops don't look like teardrops as they fall; they look like balls. And so do drops of blood. The stain that a drop of blood will eventually create can never be less than its diameter in flight. Blood in motion is not affected by the age or sex of the donor, nor will the blood alcohol level of a victim have any significant effect on the bloodstain patterns produced at the scene. A typical blood drop is .05 ml and reaches terminal velocity of about 25 feet per second in about 25 feet.

The more than twelve hundred graduates of Herb MacDonell's blood school know all this. The thirty-six students in this spring session are just learning this as they work their way through the curriculum. They will learn to consider the surface upon which the blood is found, the shape, size and distribution of the individual bloodstains, and the overall character of any large bloodstains. And just as in any good science class, they will receive this information through lectures and labs.

Class begins every morning with donuts and a lecture. Sitting in the darkened room, you can hear the soft munching of nearly forty people as they watch slide after slide of bloody crime scenes illustrating the horizontal, vertical, and high and low velocity of drops on every conceivable surface. In the afternoon lab that awaits them each day, they will get their hands dirty and really learn the stuff.

Also awaiting them is the suspense of what single thing Herb will do during this session that he's never done before, because Herb is like that. At each weeklong session, Herb presents at least one truly memorable—some might say outrageous—display. Once, for instance, he engaged his students in measuring the velocity of droplets flung off the blood-soaked, long hair of a young female volunteer.

Herb is often asked about this experiment. It arose from a case in the 1970s in Oregon in which an elderly widow, Ellen Anderson, had been severely beaten. The suspect was a woman in her twenties, Leslie Harley, who looked in on the widow, helped with housework, ran errands and acted as a companion to Anderson.

One day, Harley apparently became enraged when she learned that she would not be compensated to her liking in Mrs. Anderson's will. Her reaction was to attack the older woman with a fire poker. A review of the bloodstains revealed that attacks took place in the dining room, in the living room, on the stairway and in the bedroom. Ultimately, the widow's thick skull saved her life, and she was able to testify to the events at trial.

For its part, the defense claimed that the victim had slipped and fallen in the living room and that her head had struck the brick edge of the fireplace hearth. Harley maintained that she had helped the woman upstairs and into bed and then had begun telephoning doctors on a list kept on the bedroom desk. She claimed that the blood spatter on the ceiling of the bedroom resulted when the victim shook her head "no" over and over, rejecting one doctor and then the next whose names Harley read from the list.

Herb MacDonell had been called by the prosecution. He knew that the cast-off pattern could not have come from the victim's shaking her head. Drops resulting from even the most adamant protest would have to show a crisscross pattern from left to right if they ever reached the ceiling. These drops on the ceiling were perpendicular to a crisscross pattern and, in Herb's words, "radiated out from the area directly above the pillow with their angles of impact to the ceiling becoming more acute the farther they were from the area above the pillow. The shift in angular impact was evident by the increasing length-to-width ratio of those bloodstains that were farthest from their convergence above the pillow."

The elliptical geometry and trigonometry, of course, had to be translated to make sense to the jury. Herb knew what he had to do: It would require a model with the same length hair as the victim, but she would have to be younger and more athletic than the victim and, of course, she would have to feel no qualms about having her hair saturated with human blood.

A local nurse fit the description. So, on July 9, 1973, a small band of students made its way to the chemistry laboratory at Elmira College, armed with 35 mm and 8 mm movie cameras, 500 ml of blood, a pillow and several sheets of white cardboard. A table was set up at the correct distance below the ceiling as the bed at the crime scene. Herb massaged the blood into the nurse's hair. Then, blood-soaked and on film, she shook her head as if to say "no," over and over again, and never produced a single drop on the ceiling.

Then the model moved out of the scene, and Herb dipped a short broom handle into the blood. Rapidly raising it back over his head, he struck the pillow many times, producing patterns of blood on the classroom ceiling that were remarkably similar to those on the bedroom ceiling.

When called to the stand, Herb gave his opinion that the blood on the ceiling could not have resulted from the victim's shaking her head when her hair was soaked with blood. Herb loves to tell what happened when the defense counsel cross-examined him.

"Come now, professor, you have no basis for that opinion, have you? You certainly have never conducted experiments with a live subject whose hair was wet with blood to see how far they could shake it, have you?"

"As a matter of fact, I have done that very experiment."

Leslie Harley went to prison.

Keeping blood school fresh requires new experiments, new material. Sometimes there will be a guessing game with students who are sent off to make bloodstain patterns for the great man to identify. An apple core dipped in blood and then rolled on a page was one he figured out, as he did the bloody footprints of a leaping frog. The demonstration could involve just about anything that needs to be tested, measured, weighed, timed and eventually asked about in court. But always, with blood school comes the threat of what Herb is going to decide he needs to know about next.

The word of mouth is that this year someone is going to spit human blood on someone else.

It's Thursday morning, and it hasn't happened yet. As the thirty-six students file in and take their seats, they exchange business cards and talk about the night before. "You go out drinking?" asks one. "Scotch night. You were looking special when I left," says another. "Martini night tonight!" someone calls out, and a general wave of thumbs-up ripples through the group. A female cop shakes her head. "Oh yeah, I'm there," she says. "The thought of putting warm blood in my mouth . . ." And she stops, grimaces and takes her seat.

Looks like today's the day.

Throughout the week the group has been divided into lab pods of six, moving through fourteen experiments. By the end of the week they all will have completed each experiment and will be able to tell the origin of spatter, what kind of energy caused it, the direction from which it came, whether the victim was standing, sitting or lying down when the wound was inflicted, the movement of the assailant and victim during the encounter, the movement of both parties after the assault, and how many blows or gunshots the victim received.

Lab begins each day with students getting their buckets of blood. Lining up, each group receives human blood that has been acquired from the Red Cross after its expiration date. The containers in which the groups receive their pints vary: At table fourteen, the blood is poured into a hacked-off, one-gallon supermarket jug that once held vinegar.

It's all very matter-of-fact here: It's blood, we're going to throw it around, watch how it moves, learn something about it and that's all there is to it. No one seems to think this is the least bit odd; or at least no one is saying so—not Phyllis MacDonell, Herb's wife, who oversees an experiment at the back of the room;

not two local beat cops who stroll in off the streets of Corning for a donut and a couple of hellos and poke around a bit; not the students and not even the street person who shuffles to the glass doors, cups his hands over his eyes, peers in, smirks, backs up, collects the few discarded cans out by the soda machine and shuffles off again.

Those students not casting off, dropping or hurling blood stand around watching others do so, drinking out of the coffee mugs they've been given—the ones with BLOODSTAIN EVIDENCE INSTITUTE, CORNING, NEW YORK printed in black over the replica blood spatters mottling the white cup. The students scribble in lab manuals also spattered in the pattern of bloodstains. It would be fair to say that the place is nearly covered in blood: While they are here, people have blood on their hands, on their shoes and their shirts and on their minds. That's what they pay for and that's why they come.

In experiment number one, students are attempting to establish a reference volume of a single drop of blood, as well as its diameter in air. The first half of this experiment utilizes an ingenious syringe/pipette/clamp contraption Herb has assembled that slowly drips blood, one drop at a time, into a beaker. The second half of the experiment is designed to illustrate more practical circumstances of dropping blood by connecting a piece of glass tubing to a small funnel and then to a contraption on a volunteer's arm, with the open end pointing down at the elbow. With the clamp closed and the funnel supported, the blood is added. When the clamp is opened a slow flow of blood will stream down the arm and drip from the elbow into a ten-milliliter flared-top graduated cylinder. Counting the drops until five to ten milliliters have been collected, the students divide the total volume collected by the number of drops observed to reach the average size of a single drop.

Knowing the importance of a single drop of blood could have resulted in a conviction at the criminal trial for the murders of Nicole Brown Simpson and Ronald Goldman. In fact, if the coroner's staff at the murders had not turned over Nicole's body, we might know beyond a reasonable doubt who killed those two innocent people.

When Herb MacDonell received copies of 150 crime scene photographs from the Simpson case, he was a little disappointed— pleased to be asked to participate in the trial, but unhappy to get only the photos. Usually he requests and will be sent a scene diagram, autopsy protocol and all the technical reports that may have been generated on such things as fingerprint comparisons, firearms examinations, and hair and fiber comparisons. But he would have to wait for those.

As he reviewed the pictures, he knew that what he saw in the blood would keep him busy for a while. MacDonell was initially struck by three details: the huge amount of blood at the scene, the small area in which the murders took place, and the fact that no one had collected and analyzed the blood on Nicole's back.

Someone had bled on Nicole Brown Simpson. The evidence was right there in the photos, the blood exposed by the halter top she was wearing when she died. Nicole Brown Simpson had been stabbed and her throat slashed; the result had been a massive amount of blood loss. It had pooled everywhere around the body. But because she was facedown, it could not have flowed onto her back. The drops on her back clearly had come from someone else at the scene.

In the photographs, those drops of blood emblazoned her bare back like the arrows they could have been. It was possible, even probable, that they could have pointed to the genetic code of whoever took her life and that of her friend Ronald Goldman.

But after the drops were captured on the photographs taken by police, they were lost. Nobody lifted them from Nicole's skin to be analyzed and preserved. When the police completed their crime scene investigation, the coroner's people lifted Nicole's body and rolled her into a sheet and onto her back. They zipped her body into a bag and placed it in the morgue wagon. And as they were doing that, some of the blood leaking from her cut throat washed all the other spots of blood off her skin forever. No one thought to preserve those spots of blood and protect them by moving the body as it was—facedown. Apparently, no one at the scene understood how important they were.

The body of Nicole Brown Simpson was turned onto its back partly out of respect for the dead and partly out of convenience, but mostly out of habit. In fact, this was a case of a seemingly good habit gone bad.

One of the reasons that a body is traditionally turned on its back when moved from the scene of death is because funeral directors do not want the family and friends to have to see lividity—literally, the color of death—in the face of their loved one. Simple physics makes the red blood cells in a dead body gravitate downward, turning the dependent skin a deep maroon. This is the same settling process seen in a bag when you donate blood. The blood settles into its component parts. The front of the body, and most particularly the face, takes on a deep flush, making the embalmer's job difficult if the family is planning for the body to be viewed prior to burial. So we tend to turn bodies faceup to leave a more normal color for viewing.

That is a fine practice in cases of natural death. But at a homicide scene, this practice destroys evidence. Had Nicole's body been transported to the morgue in the position in which it was found, most likely those drops of blood—as well as fibers, prints and numerous other pieces of evidence on her back—would have been available for analysis.

MacDonell had to work with what he was given. Using a model who was the same weight and height as Nicole, he set out to re-create the lost bloodstain pattern to see what he could learn. Five photographs in particular showed the spatter. He carefully copied the pattern onto the model's exposed back. She then assumed the position in which Nicole had been found—facedown, in a black halter top, her legs and arms positioned exactly like

Nicole's. And then the blood was copied onto her back below her blond hair. It was an eerie reenactment.

Up close, individual drops of blood read like little road signs. But as the viewer stands back and looks down at a whole pattern of bloodstain evidence, the picture broadens into something more like a map of the world. And much like a journey, there is a point of origin as well as a destination.

Basic trigonometric calculations of the impact of the blood-stains are made using the length-to-width ratio of the bloodstains. Unfortunately, the Los Angeles police did not include a ruler in its crime scene photos of Nicole's back, so the actual size of the bloodstains on her back had to be estimated.

Keeping in mind that these blood spatters were not from Nicole but from someone else, it became necessary to establish where that person was when he bled onto her. Was he lying next to her, for instance? Or was he standing over her, bleeding onto her from above? To establish this, the angles of impact were metic-ulously calculated.

It took time and energy, and it all seemed very important to Herb MacDonell, especially in light of the lack of other informa-tion about the blood. But when the so-called Trial of the Century was held in Los Angeles and Herb was called to the stand, no one asked him about that meticulous research and its findings. It was never requested at trial.

This happens a lot. The expert is ready to go, but no one asks the right question. MacDonell says he'd do the same amount of work tomorrow on any blood case, as would anyone he teaches, because at blood school it is understood that to read a crime scene you read the blood, drop by precious drop. And that is why, in Corning, New York, you start at experiment number one: estab-lishing a reference volume of a single drop of blood along with its diameter in the air. Because a spatter analyst is only as good as what he or she can read in a single drop of blood.

In experiment two, students measure vertical blood spatter in relation to the distance the blood falls and the target surface covered. It's a fairly tame exercise, involving a plumb line, a tape measure and ten drops of blood hitting a target surface. The third experiment makes a convincing argument that any attempt to describe the character of a spot of blood is absolutely meaningless without considering the surface texture of where it lands. Students take turns emptying droppers full of blood onto newspaper, paper towel, cloth, glass, floor tile, blotter and wood. The terms start to change here: The big drop is the "central bloodstain" and those little marks around it, but not connected to it, are "satellite spatter" and "spines" that streak out from the central stain.

Moving on to experiment four, one finds a table of nine different clipboards mounted at ten-degree increments. On each there is a variation of the elliptical nature of blood spots falling at an angle onto flat surfaces. The message is clear: As the impact angle decreases from 90 degrees to 10 degrees, the shape of the bloodstain changes from a circle to an ellipse.

In experiment number five, it looks as though someone ran from the room bleeding. Even to the untrained eye, the blood drops strewn along the paper on the floor seem to be pointing toward the door. This is a test of horizontal motion on bloodstain: The more rapid the horizontal motion, the more the breakup of the drops in the direction of movement. Frequently, a smaller droplet will be thrown off in a backlash from its parent drop. These are described as "tadpoles" and "castoffs," which travel in the same direction as the original drop.

Splashed blood is observed at table six, while projected blood is the subject of experiment seven. A large PVC and paper roll box contains experiment number eight. In the box stands a police officer, one of MacDonell's students, dressed entirely in medical scrubs, complete with a footsie (medical bootie) on his head. These are the instructions for the experiment: "Dip one end of either a metal rod or wooden stick into freshly stirred blood, covering it thoroughly. Allow some of the blood to drain off and then simulate a swinging or chopping action. Care must be taken that the assault weapon is swung in an arc, which will confine the cast-off blood so it strikes the 'cocoon.' Some blood will be cast off during the downward swing onto the forward (vertical) targets. Mark the corresponding stains to the mechanism that created them, and repeat the experiment with different objects and varying numbers of speeds and swings. Study these patterns and identify the sequence of blows on both the overhead and vertical targets." In other words, simulate hacking, hammering and beating someone to death.

Experiment nine studies medium-velocity blood spatter by slapping five milliliters of well-mixed human blood in a "medium-velocity impact apparatus," a.k.a. the "rat trap." Spatter of this type consists of small droplets resulting from chopping, beating, stabbing or impact from an object moving at a velocity of approximately 25 feet per second. These blood drops will be larger than those coming from high-velocity impact, which is tested in experiment ten.

You can tell when experiment ten is up and running because it is always preceded by the shout "Fire in the hall!" which is immediately followed by a gunshot from a .22-caliber rifle set securely into a box, facing a blood-soaked target, behind which is a bullet trap. Every few minutes comes another shout, another rifle shot and another set of notations scribbled in the lab book.

MacDonell's ability to understand the effect of a single gunshot on blood helped Susie Mowbray get out of prison recently, after wrongly serving nine years of a life sentence for the death of her husband.

The case began in Brownsville, Texas, in October 1987, when William Mowbray, a prominent Brownsville Cadillac dealer, was killed in his bed by a single contact gunshot wound to his right temple. In November, MacDonell received a call from the local prosecutor, asking him to look at some evidence. Two days later, a team of prosecutors came to Corning.

The evidence was a long-sleeved, white nightgown Susie was wearing the night of the shooting. MacDonell was convinced it showed much more to exonerate her than to suggest she ever shot her husband. A stereomicroscopic examination of the nightgown revealed no trace of blood anywhere on the garment.

MacDonell keeps very precise notes. Books of them, in fact, line the lower-level office in his home. Flipping through any of them gives the reader the sense that this man misses nothing: The time of every call is written down—the first call from the prosecutor in the Mowbray case came at 3:43 P.M., for instance—as are the case number and every observation made.

A tight contact gunshot wound—meaning one in which the muzzle of the weapon is pressed firmly against the skin—usually creates a stellate, or star-shaped, wound, which occurs when the expanding gases leaving the muzzle enter the space under the skin but above the bone, stretching and rupturing the skin. The skin tears away from the bullet hole's entrance as it reaches its elasticity. The hole shows radial lacerations and appears starlike in its geometry.

MacDonell wanted to view the Mowbray murder scene, so on December 1, 1987, he traveled to Brownsville. He found very fine bloodstains on the bed's headboard that allowed him to locate the origin of the high-velocity back-spatter on the bed. It was on the side of the dead man. The sheet was bloodstained by back-spattered blood. And if there was blood on the sheet and Susie had shot him at close range, didn't it stand to reason that blood would also appear on her nightgown? Susie had not had time to change her nightgown before the couple's daughter ran into the room immediately after hearing the gunshot. The lack of blood on Susie Mowbray's nightgown led MacDonell to conclude firmly that it was unlikely that the nightgown was in close proximity to the victim and that therefore the death was more probably a suicide.

This apparently was not what the prosecution wanted to hear. So they found another witness who sprayed the nightgown with luminol and testified to seeing luminescent spots when the garment was viewed in a dark room. He testified that he identified and measured the spots, determining they were high-velocity impact blood spatter.

MacDonell was never called to testify and lost track of the case, as happens in many of the cases when he is dismissed. The file went to dead storage in his barn until six years and eight months later when he received a telephone call from Robert Ford, a defense attorney in Fort Worth, Texas, who told him that Susie Mowbray had long ago been convicted of murder and sentenced to life imprisonment. Ford was working on an appeal.

At the habeas corpus hearing, the judge determined that the testimony that had sent Mowbray away was scientifically invalid because it was uncorroborated and found that the prosecutors had knowingly suppressed from the jury MacDonell's report stating that Bill Mowbray's death was likely a suicide. Further, the judge observed that Susie Mowbray likely would have been acquitted if MacDonell had testified. A new trial was ordered.

The second trial of Susie Mowbray began on January 12, 1998. This time MacDonell took the stand. Another witness who had not made it into court the first time, a local banker, testified that a distraught Bill Mowbray had come into his office two or three days before the shooting and said that he would kill himself if the banker did not make him a large personal loan.

Susie Mowbray was acquitted. She had served nine years in prison for a murder she didn't commit. During an interview after the trial, the county's chief felony prosecutor said he was "disappointed" with the verdict and acknowledged he had made a tactical error when, in court, he asked the key defense witness his fee for working with the defense team. Herb MacDonell had replied under oath that he was working for free to right a wrong.

Students moving through the lab experiments at blood school hear the stories, and they seem to help the students focus while their gloved hands are awash in blood. Four experiments remain. A motor-driven blood spatter device is included in experiment eleven, where spot size versus horizontal projection is measured. At table twelve is the odd assortment of wigs, cotton T-shirts, a fire poker, some hammers, shoes and a newel post, all of which get dipped in blood and wiped, tapped, hammered, dragged and rolled across, along and on top of large sheets of white paper to record their transfer patterns.

Experiment thirteen is about volume—bringing us from experiment one, analyzing a single drop of blood, to here, where blood has gushed. By now you have seen just about everything there is to see and are ready to test what you know by reporting to Phyllis MacDonell, who sits at experiment fourteen. She oversees a mini crime scene and will answer questions and hand out necessary documents (autopsy reports, crime scene reports) to the inquisitive law enforcement officers who try to reconstruct what happened when a bottle of Jack Daniel's, an unhappy couple and a rifle came together one night in front of a grandfather clock. Phyllis sits coolly by the scaled-down living room that resembles a wing of a large dollhouse from hell.

Herb MacDonell, meanwhile, is tuning up his video camera and finding the best vantage spot in the room.

"Paul Kish had a case like this," he says, as the occupants of the room begin to gather, "where the pathologist testified that stains as small as were found couldn't come from a nose and mouth. But Paul was of the opinion that they could.

"He has done this himself. The blood that is blown, wheezed, sneezed out of your mouth looks like gunshot, looks like high velocity. So, after he did the experiment and brought it into court, the guy had to back down. You have to know."

And that brings us to show time.

As MacDonell focuses his video camera, a big cop in the corner is wrestling with what looks like a large piece of cloth. As he struggles with the straps, it seems that this might be this cop's first time in an apron. He is talking to no one in particular, as a collection of colleagues forms around him.

"I'm gonna get shit all over me," he says, tugging hard at the garment.

"No," calls out MacDonell from behind his camera, his eye pressed firmly against the viewfinder, the tape rolling, "it'll be blood."

Nervous laughter. Two law enforcement agents, both women, are as far away as they can be, sitting near the donuts at a desk, not moving toward the group. Called to by a colleague, they wave him off.

"No thanks," says one.

Three of the taller participants are lining the wall with brown paper while someone rushes in clutching a brand-new package of Fruit of the Loom T-shirts. A value pack.

The big guy, having finally subdued the apron, approaches a chair near a phlebotomist who is ready to draw blood with her carry-all of syringes, rubber tourniquets and vacutainers. Another cop volunteers to get into one of the new, white T-shirts.

The blood is drawn from the big cop. MacDonell is taping. Several cops turn away. Others lift their cameras, flashes ready to go.

Paul Kish, MacDonell's longtime assistant, talks to the cop in the apron, who is now standing before him, holding a vacutainer of his own warm blood.

It's Kish's experiment, really. The big guy in the apron has a case like this coming to trial, and he wants to be ready. Kish is telling the cop what to do.

"We want you to expirate over and over onto paper," he says, pointing to the paper on the wall. Kish stands holding sheets of white cardboard, which he will hold up as a target. The brown paper behind it will catch anything that misses the target.

The cop in the apron tips the vacutainer to his lips as the camera flashes start to pop. He fills his mouth with the blood and then steps up to the paper held before him.

"Blow."

He does.

Another white cardboard goes up.

Blood has never looked so red as it does on the white cardboard.

"Blow."

"How you doing?"

He nods "okay."

The other cop, who put the new T-shirt on over his scrubs, is smiling. He becomes the next target. Someone thinks to hold a piece of white cardboard over his face as the cop in the apron takes another mouthful, steps up to his colleague and blows blood all over his chest. It's a good idea they covered the man's face because the cardboard is instantly spattered.

"Blow."

"Blow."

"That's it," says Kish, taking the vacutainer. "You can't ingest anymore."

"Turn around! Turn around!" someone yells and as the first cop does, cameras flash, catching the blood dripping down from a corner of his mouth, running down his chin and onto his throat.

"Stick out your tongue!"

More camera flashes.

"Don't swallow," says Kish, as he directs the cop out of the room.

When the resulting spatter is examined, the fine blood droplets and the pattern they leave give the appearance of a high-velocity gunshot back-spatter. Before witnessing this experiment, the observers could have easily mistaken that spatter for what might land on a close-up shooter. Conversely, if someone shot himself, and you ran up to help him as he was coughing and dying, you could end up with that same type of spatter on your shirt and be accused of being the shooter. Knowing what is there could be the difference between a conviction and an exoneration. You'd have to hope that someone who had been to blood school would be on the case.

Minutes later, the cop in the apron is back, having rinsed his mouth and smoked a Vantage from the pack he carries in one hand. In his other is a bottle of apple juice from which he is taking long, deep swigs.

Snack time. Everyone goes back to the donuts.

"I like to do things that are challenging to people's thought process," says MacDonell, getting a cup of coffee.

"And I encourage them to save the targets they make. Save the things that blood spatters on and preserve them, and you've got something no one can dispute. You don't have to say you read it in a book: It's called firsthand knowledge. They can say you did it wrong, of course, but they cannot say you didn't do it."

He looks out over his classroom at the Union Hall, blood everywhere, people eating donuts, a gun firing. And he smiles.

"So, the next time some attorney says to one of these students, 'Aw, come on, you've never actually done experiments on live models to see what patterns human blood spraying out of a mouth really look like, have you?' they can say, 'Well, actually, I have.'"

Three
WITNESS

Long before there was any talk of diamond-inlaid handcuffs, séances or "chasing the dragon," there was a phone call. That's how a case usually runs: from the mundane to the remarkable; from what happens in every case (the phone call) to what makes a case unique (jewel-studded sex toys and a séance to raise a dead man who, in life, liked inhaling the smoke of toasting heroin). The phone call to the office may bring a request to do or attend an autopsy, review another medical examiner's autopsy report, look at some slides or read a toxicology record. Eventually it will lead to the details of how someone lived and how he came to die.

This is how we move between the cause of death and the manner of death. They are two different things. Related, but different. The cause of death—what killed someone—is usually a quite simple and straightforward science. Most cops on the scene can point to it—"Look, Doc, two bullet holes"—and usually they are right.

But the manner of death is riddled with details. This is where you find the range of human imagination from the diamond-studded handcuffs to autoeroticism's elaborate pulleys and knots, which were meant to untie, but didn't. Whereas the cause of death can be a blunt trauma, the manner of death can be an accident from a fall, a suicide from a jump or a homicide from cheating on your fortune-teller and getting whacked with her crystal ball. As a body lies on the morgue table, the impact to the head—the cause of death—might look like it came from a bowling ball or even a fishbowl, but the story of who betrayed whom, and where and when the body was found, would tell the manner of death and lead to its classification as a homicide.

The questions the forensic pathologist deals with are what caused the death and how it happened. Notice, there is no discussion of who did it. I don't do that. That's not my job to decide. That's the job of the police, the prosecutor and ultimately the jury. I determine what happened, not whodunit.

The cause and manner of death fit neatly together. But while one may lead to the other, they can come to investigators in either order: A dead man with two bullets in him may turn up with no clues, or someone may be reported missing from a home in which the living room is pocked with bullet holes and spattered with blood.

You can get one without the other, or you can get neither, as happened on August 6, 1930, when Judge Joseph F. Crater told friends he was going to the theater and disappeared from the streets of New York without a trace. He is still referred to by many as the most famous missing man in America. Theories abound. Earlier that day, the judge had removed large quantities of paperwork from his office and had cashed a sizable check. Those details seem to point to someone who wanted to disappear: purge your files, get some cash, create an alibi. But to date there is no known reason for him to do so. And there is still no body, no manner and no cause of death.

The same was the case with Jimmy Hoffa, the longtime Teamsters Union boss, who others maintain is America's most infamous missing man. He certainly still draws a crowd, as he did on July 30, 1995, when two thousand mourners (including one member of the United States Congress) turned out to remember the man, who was officially declared dead in 1982. The service was held twenty years to the day after he disappeared from the parking lot of the Machus Red Fox restaurant in Bloomfield Township, outside Detroit, Michigan. No body was ever found, and no manner or cause of death was ever determined.

The medical examiner has certain options if no body is ever found, and declaring someone dead without a body is something medical examiners are occasionally asked to do. Such a declaration can be made after some time—as it was seven years following the disappearance of Hoffa—but it is always based on the circumstances.

On July 17, 1996, TWA Flight 800, a Boeing 747 bound for Paris, exploded shortly after takeoff from New York's JFK Airport, killing all 230 people on board. The medical examiners on the scene (of whom I was one) worked day and night to identify bodies. The issue arose as to how to issue a death certificate if no body was found. It was decided by Dr. Charles Wetli, the chief medical examiner of Suffolk County, that we would have to work from the passenger list as well as from interviews with family members to establish whether the person did indeed board the plane, and whether he or she was seen again after the plane departed. The airline roster is more reliable with international flights than with domestic ones because passports must be shown. Also, it is not uncommon in domestic disasters to have one or two people traveling under a different name.

As we struggled through the investigation of TWA 800, we agreed to issue death certificates for the missing at the end of the search. That turned out to be unnecessary: In the end, all the bodies were identified, some from very small pieces of tissue aided by the new DNA technologies. But a judgment had been made that the circumstances alone would have dictated such a declaration.

Declaring a person dead based on something even as individual as a tooth is difficult: People sometimes lose teeth. It's the same with fingers and, in some instances, even hands. A half century ago, a young man in Boston faced the charge of murdering his girlfriend, who he claimed had simply wandered away from him in a wooded area and then disappeared. When a hand was found in those woods, he was indicted. But during his trial the estranged girlfriend walked into the courtroom—both hands intact.

The hand, it turned out, belonged to a bear that had been skinned for its fur. Bear paws on X ray are anatomically very similar to human hands. (Nowadays, of course, DNA analysis could identify the species of the hand.)

Identification becomes a matter of judgment for medical examiners and judges. Hands do not a dead body make, and courts have been disinclined to rule someone dead when only a tooth or a hand is found. But a whole jaw may be different, as is, of course, a torso.

Jimmy Hoffa was declared dead because his family requested that declaration and because of the story—the circumstantial evidence—that he had, in fact, disappeared under mysterious circumstances. Is it possible that he is alive and well and playing cards with Elvis? It is possible. But in my professional role as an expert, I would testify on the stand that to a reasonable degree of medical certainty he is not.

Sometimes the manner and cause of death appear to be complete with little to question: a body, a scene and a story to go with it. But such a neat package can lead to all kinds of assumptions. Assumptions can be wrong—and frequently are. And that was so in the case of Ted Binion, whose death involved the jeweled handcuffs and the smoke of tar heroin.

Lonnie Ted Binion was found dead on the floor of his million-dollar Las Vegas home on September 17, 1998. The next-day headline in the *Las Vegas Review-Journal* trumpeted, "Ted Binion, Troubled Gambling Figure, Dies," with this subhead: "After a life of tumult, a former gambling executive's body is found next to an empty prescription bottle." It hardly sounded like a homicide.

The story had begun to form at 4:05 P.M. on the day Binion died, when Sandy Murphy, his live-in girlfriend, dialed 911 and screamed for help. Paramedics were unable to revive Binion, and the police who were called to the scene seemed to accept what Murphy said—that it was a drug overdose and that she had found him there on the floor.

They were dead wrong, as cops in such circumstances sometimes are. This happens all the time. Regular police precincts usually send out their experienced homicide squads only when there has been a reported homicide; their least experienced officers protect the scene when the death is reported as natural. But an experienced homicide detective can see through a staged scene. Despite national attention given to such cases as the murder of JonBenet Ramsey, we have changed little about the initial police response to the scene of a death. In the JonBenet case, the initial call to the police reporting a kidnapping resulted in certain assumptions that led to the now-infamous destruction of evidence.

No homicide detective was sent to the scene of Ted Binion's death. Sandy Murphy told the responding police a story that matched the evidence: an empty bottle of Xanax, but no suicide note, next to the body of a known heroin user whose life had spun out of control. Police recorded that, along with Murphy's reference to Binion as her "husband" and the fact that she was "hysterical," screaming, "He's not breathing! He's not breathing!"

The day after the death, the local newspaper related the story of the dead man's life. Reporters and cops alike knew about his ties to organized crime and his long-admitted heroin addiction, both of which contributed to his losing his gambling license as well as the ownership of one of Las Vegas's oldest establishments, Binion's Horseshoe, the family hotel and casino that is the site of the World Series of Poker.

It was a pure Las Vegas story, complete with a promiscuous start, a glittery midsection and a tragic finale: Two people on the outs find each other in a topless bar, live the high life together, and then one dies. It all seemed to make perfect sense.

The absence of a homicide detective from a murder scene means that there is no one present who is skilled in knowing how to protect the crime scene; no one to poke around the story being told by whoever found the body. Instead, all too often, the story is told, the body is removed and assumptions of innocence are born. And as soon as assumptions are made, trace evidence gets trampled.

Thinking you know what you are looking for is bad enough. Then you miss only the obvious. But history has proven that things get much worse when police officers assume that they are not dealing with a homicide and therefore are not supposed to be scouring the place for evidence. Then, they step all over it.

Many people feel that this is what happened in the O.J. Simpson case. As soon as the cops at the scene saw Nicole was murdered, knowing, as they did, the history of domestic violence between the estranged couple, the investigators assumed the killer was Simpson, figured there would be a quick confession and took less care than they should have in identifying, collecting, handling and preserving the evidence.

When I worked in the Office of Chief Medical Examiner of New York City from 1960 until 1985, I visited thousands of death scenes and saw an awful lot of trace evidence. These days I have a more diverse life. In private practice, I work as a forensic pathologist available for consultation, and I mostly review photographs and reports—which are evidence, but not fresh—that are mailed to me after I get that first phone call. Then, if I pursue the case, I will look at everything that is available.

As the co-director of the Medico-Legal Investigations Unit of the New York State Police, where I have served since 1985, and as the forensic pathologist for Dutchess County, New York, I still occasionally travel to crime scenes.

Most of the calls I get in my private practice come from prosecutors, police, defense lawyers or distraught family members. Often the request is made for me to re-autopsy a body following a hospital death or a cause of death determination that the family simply cannot accept. This often happens with suicides. People don't like to believe their family members may have committed suicide, so they want a re-investigation. And sometimes they are correct.

A few years ago, a bright, successful, talented, popular Ivy League student was found hanging in the attic of his dormitory building at school. The medical examiner's office determined it was suicide. But this didn't make sense to the parents: They were a close, loving family and had detected no suggestion that the young man had been depressed.

Upon reviewing the case, I, too, disagreed with the medical examiner's findings. The boy had been experimenting in the world of autoeroticism. He would partially hang himself while masturbating and supposedly would experience heightened orgasm. This time he had passed out and hanged to death. I thought the family would find this to be more upsetting, but I was surprised to learn that they could accept their son's dying as a result of sexual experimentation. They couldn't accept his dying from suicide. This realization has helped me a lot over the years in dealing with families in cases of suicide.

There is a presumption against suicide in the courts. County medical examiners come up against this all the time and have to prove that someone did, in fact, intend to kill himself and was, in fact, successful in doing so. It can be difficult to prove, especially when families challenge a cause of death finding that will exclude an insurance claim, as often happens if someone commits suicide within the two-year exclusionary period after taking the policy.

Early in my career, I was brought into court to testify about a woman I had autopsied and found to have taken more than thirty sleeping pills. In my opinion, that could only have been done intentionally. I classified her death as suicide.

But an expert psychiatrist testified for the defense that the dead woman had not been depressed. He said that on the night in question, she was tired and took some sleeping pills, after which she fell partially asleep and then developed a condition called automatism: She woke up, forgot she had taken the pills and took another two. She did this—wake up, take two pills, fall partially asleep, wake up, take two pills, fall partially asleep—fifteen times, the psychiatrist testified.

There was a double indemnity, $200,000 insurance policy on the line: If her death had been accidental, the payment would have been $400,000; if it was suicide, it was nothing. In this case, the family had brought a civil action against the insurance company for nonpayment of the policy.

It is my experience that judges tend to allow all sorts of testimony in cases like this because the parents, spouse and children of the deceased are typically sitting in the front row of the courtroom every day. It has a tremendous effect. Juries, too, see the suffering family. They don't want to punish the children for their parents' behavior, and they equally don't care about insurance companies. And so they tend to side with the plaintiffs—the potential recipients of the payment.

Civil cases like these become battles of experts, because all parties can afford to pay the fees: The plaintiff's lawyer is operating on a contingency basis; if he wins, he gets paid, but if he loses, the family pays nothing. The insurance companies are rich and can pay experts plenty to protect their assets. Despite the way it is represented on television and despite the impression left by the O.J. Simpson case, most criminal cases do not include testimony by experts, for the simple reason that most defendants are typically poor, have inexperienced lawyers and cannot afford experts.

It's not that O.J. Simpson had too much expert assistance; it's that poor people have too little. In fact, one of the many problems with the death penalty that has only recently been brought to light is that most defendants do not have the money to hire such expert witnesses, and the court allowances do not give them enough to do so.

When a big tobacco company is being sued, the plaintiff's attorney taking on the case knows up front whether there will be a lot of money for expert testimony. Without that, the lawyer would not take the case. A large percentage of civil litigation is done by contingency. So a lot more attention is paid to the facts in a civil trial, in which money is involved, than in a criminal trial, when only the life of a human being is at stake. So, if you want to see an array of experts—forensic engineers, forensic climatologists, forensic linguists, forensic geologists—go to civil court.

In the overdose insurance case, I had done the autopsy and had testified in court. I was very young and inexperienced and took it personally when the jury ruled against my finding and in favor of the family. I felt that they did not believe me and that it was somehow my fault that justice was not being done. I felt they had ruled against *me*.

Over the years I have learned not to take these things personally. From the moment someone calls, a process is set into motion that could go any number of ways. My impact on the case can be only as good as the science I do and how well I explain it in court.

The phone call alerting me to the Ted Binion case came to my private practice. It was from Tom Dillard, a former Las Vegas homicide detective turned private investigator. He said he had heard of me and asked if I would review an autopsy report and a toxicology report. That was all he had. That, and a backstory with all the seedy facets of film noir.

The characters were Sandy Murphy, Lonnie Ted Binion and Rick Tabish: the ex-stripper, her millionaire boyfriend and her secret lover. Spiking the drama were the facts that the lover was in serious financial debt and that he was arrested right after the death for digging up the late boyfriend's buried treasure in the desert; that the boyfriend was thirty years older than the ex-stripper; and that he had used heroin for fifteen years, but didn't shoot it, snort it or smoke it. He chased the dragon.

It is a method of heroin use popular in China and other countries where heroin is very cheap, but a method seldom used in America. Chasing the dragon involves heating tar heroin on foil and inhaling the resulting white smoke. This smoke curls upward and looks to some like the tail or the breath of a dragon. Other than geographic difference, chasing the dragon is distinguished by another exclusive quality: In this country, at least, no one has ever reportedly died from this means of heroin use.

One night Binion called his lawyer and instructed him to take Sandy Murphy out of the will in which he had left her his $900,000 house and $300,000 in cash. "If she doesn't kill me tonight," he added. Apparently she did. Within days her lover, Rick Tabish, was found by law enforcement officers in the desert digging up Binion's stash of silver bullion and coins, valued at $5 million.

Clark County Medical Examiner Lary Simms had been on the job only a few weeks when the body of Ted Binion turned up on his autopsy table. Despite Binion's known heroin addiction, one could not assume that he died of an overdose. And so toxicological tests were run. They revealed Xanax, an anti-anxiety drug that Binion was known to take when trying to stay off heroin. But the Xanax appeared to be present in a larger dose than could be taken accidentally. Also found was morphine, a breakdown product of heroin. Because of these findings, along with what was known of the history and circumstances, Simms determined the cause of death to be a drug overdose and the manner of death to be homicide.

The Clark County Medical Examiner's office contacted another medical examiner in Reno to review the matter. She confirmed Simms's conclusions. Her report was typed up and sent to Clark County.

But all this had taken several months, during which time Binion's family had grown uncomfortable with the lack of a determination of homicide. And in the interim it had emerged that Murphy and Tabish were lovers.

Tom Dillard, hired by Binion's suspicious family, sent me the report from the Reno medical examiner. At the time of his initial call, the reports from the Clark County Medical Examiner's office had not yet been released. After reviewing the Reno report, I sent a one-page letter to Mr. Dillard stating that I agreed with Dr. Simms's conclusions on the basis of the information I had reviewed. I had not yet seen the original documents from Clark County nor any photographs. I followed up the letter with a call to Dillard and said that since I agreed with Dr. Simms, "I guess you don't need me anymore."

That is the way it usually goes: I concur with the findings of the local medical examiner and I don't get called to the witness stand. Or, conversely, I disagree with the local examiner and I don't get called to the witness stand. In fact, in the great majority of cases in which I consult, I do not get called to testify. Often the accused is apprised of the outside findings (mine) and then pleads guilty to a lesser charge. Then no one gets called to the witness stand, because no one goes to court.

But every once in a while you go the distance.

Tom Dillard told me that David Rogers and David Wall, the prosecutors in the Binion case, were a little concerned about the length of time it was taking Dr. Simms to establish the cause and manner of death. Even though I was technically employed by the family, not the DA, the prosecutor wanted me to back up Simms's findings at the preliminary hearing. A preliminary hearing is like an open grand jury, where evidence is presented to a judge, but no jury, and witnesses are both examined and cross-examined. Then a decision is rendered whether or not to indict someone.

For that role, I thought I should do a more thorough review of the material. I needed to see it all—the autopsy photos, the tissue samples taken at autopsy, the clothing of the deceased, as well as any police reports and other documentation. And I needed to visit the scene of the death.

I flew into Las Vegas the day before the preliminary hearing and was met by Tom Dillard, who took me to the medical examiner's office.

The first things I saw when I got there were the photos. Right away I thought something was wrong. Simms seemed to sense this and grew visibly uncomfortable with my presence. It's odd, because I enjoy having people review my work. That way, if there is a misinterpretation of the evidence, it is caught long before trial. He didn't seem to agree.

The pictures of the dead man's eyes revealed distinct petechial hemorrhages inside the lower lids, suggesting compression of the neck.

Petechial hemorrhages are capillaries that have ruptured because of pressure. The circulatory system consists of arteries, veins and capillaries. Simply put, arteries pump blood out from the heart, the blood continues into the capillaries, where it provides oxygen to the cells and then continues into the veins, which bring the deoxygenated blood back to the heart. If pressure is put on the neck, the blood backs up and the capillaries, which are the weakest part of the vascular system, can rupture; this sometimes happens when you sneeze too hard, causing a blood spot to appear in your eye. It takes sixty to seventy pounds of pressure to collapse an artery, but only five pounds to collapse a vein.

In suffocation, the pressure is primarily on the nose and mouth, not on the neck, and usually you do not see petechiae. However, when a person struggles, this often inadvertently leads to pressure on the neck, as well. A finding of strangulation is a subtle one, and suffocation is much more rare than strangulation. Of the thousands of autopsies I've performed since 1960, only a few dozen were found to be adult deaths resulting from suffocation.

Dr. Simms and I differed on whether there was congestion in the capillaries in the eyelids or actual rupture of capillaries. However, we didn't differ on the presence of significant bruising or rubbing of the skin around the mouth. We also both noted the presence of small, circular bruises that looked like button imprints on the dead man's chest and another large bruise to the front of the ribs. There were also interesting bruises on both of the dead man's wrists—small, round marks, the type most associated with handcuffs.

While Simms and I agreed on the presence of all of these bruises—they were right there on the photos—we would come to differ about what they meant.

Simms had rightly taken tissue samples from various parts of the body and preserved them in formaldehyde. These samples are normally taken from every organ in the body—the heart, each lung, the pancreas, each kidney, the brain, the liver, adrenal glands, and so forth. To do the best job, samples of any bruises should be taken at autopsy, as well. In this case, only some had been taken at autopsy.

Looking at the photos again, I saw one bruise in particular that interested me. Thankfully, a tissue sample of that one existed. It was a bruise over the lower ribs, and by the looks of it, it could not have formed more than just shortly before the time of death. This suspicion was confirmed under the microscope.

At the time the body is bruised—say, a punch in the eye at a boxing match—little capillaries are ruptured and bleed, resulting in what we call a black-and-blue mark. Left to its natural devices, the body will respond to that bruise within an hour. Its first response is to hemorrhage. Then, after an hour or so, it sends in the white cells, or inflammatory cells. A hemorrhage without this response is called a bland hemorrhage, and we know it is fresh. If the person dies before an hour has passed since the bruise formed, there will be no response, and all that can be seen under the microscope at autopsy is fresh red blood cells.

If Ted Binion had lived for an hour after this bruise, I would have seen cells from the body trying to repair itself when I looked at his tissue samples under the microscope. There were none.

This is very important to the forensic pathologist, but less so to the hospital pathologist, whose job it is to notice how we die, not necessarily when. When I was a resident doctor at Bellevue Hospital, most deaths were recorded as having occurred at about 6 A.M., when the nurses made medication rounds and found the bodies of anyone who had died during the night. The time of death did not matter in these patients, so times of death were listed as the time where the bodies were found.

I paused to reflect: If I can't see the body's normal repair process, I know the man died within an hour of being bruised. This could speak to a struggle. But could it speak to cardiopulmonary resuscitation (CPR)? Did someone trying to resuscitate him cause this bruising? Was this a case of death by friendly fire?

A friendly bruise or a hostile one—how do you know?

Many months later, in his closing argument at the murder trial, John Momot, Sandy Murphy's defense attorney, said, "She loves him. He loves heroin, and the heroin loves no one." It was a good defense. It had been Sandy Murphy's story from the start.

It was what she told the emergency medical technicians and then the cops when they rushed to the million-dollar home of Ted Binion. It was what Sandy Murphy had told anybody and everybody who would listen for a good long time before her boyfriend turned up dead. When she told it to the cops at the scene of his death, they believed her. It sure looked like an overdose. He was a known heroin user and had been for fifteen years. Las Vegas is, after all, a small town; everybody knew that Binion had lost his gambling license, the ownership of his family's famous casino, as well as a long marriage because of the drugs. It all made sense.

Until the autopsy.

When CPR is performed on a living person, it can result in extensive bruising. Sternal rubbing, pounding on the chest, flipping over a person struggling for life—all of these may cause bruises to the body. There can be a lot of breaking of blood vessels in an effort to prolong life. A large hemorrhage, or bruise, develops when the heart is still beating and pumping blood. If the person is already dead when CPR is started, there may be some bruising, but it will be slight. This is because any bleeding will be passive, since the heart has stopped. That does not mean there is no blood in the body, only that it has little pressure behind it. Imagine cutting a garden hose when the water is turned off: You'll get a little leakage of water flowing passively. Cut the hose when the water is on, however, and the active pressure will make it spurt.

As I looked at the pictures and the tissues of Ted Binion, the story envisioned by Dr. Simms began to unravel for me. It was a troubling development. I had been flown out to support the conclusion that Ted Binion had died of a forced ingestion of a combination of Xanax and heroin. Suddenly that was not my opinion. I couldn't swear to that. And I wouldn't.

Usually if I am coming in on the same side and there are differing opinions, we talk about them freely: He sees this, I see that, but we are both there to advocate for the dead, for justice. We are both forensic scientists, so really we are on the side of the science. Any forensic scientist who feels that he must advocate for the side standing in the room is going to get into trouble.

This applies even when doing the job as the county medical

examiner. The position does not require you to side with the prosecution: You must always ally yourself only with the science. The job a person holds must not influence a scientific finding.

Dr. Simms and I ran into trouble when I said that what he had listed in his report as congested vessels in the eye looked to me like petechial hemorrhages. He said that he had his opinion and that I could have mine, and that he didn't think it was appropriate to discuss it further. But he did make all the records, photos and samples available to me.

While looking at the original reports, I realized that there was something amiss. Comparing them to the copies I had been sent and had reviewed, I saw that the report typed at the medical examiner's office in Reno—a copy of which I had originally been sent—had an error in the toxicology report. Instead of listing the Xanax found in Mr. Binion in nanograms per milliliter, it had been listed in milligrams, which is a million times more. Instead of typing "ng," someone had typed "mg."

It was from this information that I had drawn my original conclusion that the amount in the body was a lethal level. In fact, what was found in Mr. Binion was a therapeutic level and one that can be easily tolerated by most people.

As a medical examiner I know that at any time some other professional may come and review my work. He might be someone come to back me up or someone from the opposite side brought in to review things. The family, in particular, has a right to review what we've done, which is one of the reasons we contemporaneously document everything we see. We dictate, take photographs and X rays, make microscopic slides: Everything we do, in fact, is done so that another person can come in and make an independent assessment, not relying on us. In the old days we said, "Trust me." There were few photos, no clothing analysis, and no independent judgment. And that's how lots of mistakes were made.

When we got outside the lab where I had reviewed Dr. Simms's findings and the data, I knew what I had to say. "This doesn't make sense now," I told Dillard. "I don't agree with Simms."

Dillard didn't look pleased.

There are five manners of death: accident, suicide, homicide, natural and undetermined. Dr. Simms had concluded Binion had died as a homicide due to overdose. But the facts, in my opinion, indicated that the levels of the drugs in Binion's system were not high enough to kill him. So while it may, in fact, have been a homicide, I told Dillard, it was unlikely that the homicide was caused by overdose. I based this finding on several things.

First, in my opinion you don't die from chasing the dragon. Certainly not in the United States. After thousands of heroin autopsies in New York City, several trips to Hong Kong (where heroin use by chasing the dragon is very popular) and an extensive search of the pertinent medical literature, I have not been able to identify a single such death. That makes the chances of Binion's dying this way very small—possible, but highly unlikely.

Then there was the fact that there were no injection marks on Binion's body. That means that not only did he not shoot the heroin but that no one injected him with it against his will. So how did the heroin get into his system?

Experience has taught me that it is very hard to force someone else to swallow enough of anything to cause death. I once had a case where a man had pointed a gun at his wife and said, "Swallow," as she downed what he thought would be enough sleeping pills to kill her. They weren't and they didn't. He was a physician, and even he didn't get it right. He had forced her to take enough medication to make her pass out, but she recovered and helped convict him.

Sometimes, of course, people die accidentally after taking drugs, especially as a result of drug interaction, when the combination of two or more drugs causes a reaction in the patient that one drug alone would not have caused.

The first photocopied autopsy report I had received and reviewed had indicated an amount of Xanax in Binion that he could not have taken by accident, and as a result, I ruled out accidental death, which left me with suicide or homicide.

Now, with the presence of the petechiae, the bruises on the chest, the freshness of those bruises, the circumstances of the death and the toxicological results, it was my opinion that although there were drugs in Binion's system, they were not sufficient to cause death. They were, I was convinced, just an incidental finding. I agreed that the manner of death was homicide. But I believed that the cause of death was suffocation.

As I was telling Dillard this, I could see that it was causing him concern. He had wanted my opinion. But he hadn't expected this one. He excused himself and went to call the DA, David Rogers. He too, it turned out, was concerned by this new and surprising opinion.

The preliminary hearing was scheduled for the next day; I had been flown in to act as backup witness to Simms. I wondered whether they wanted to put me back on the plane to New York with a big, "Thank you, but no thank you."

Dillard, Rogers, Wall and I went out to dinner to go over my findings. At 6 P.M. on the eve of the preliminary hearing, we sat down to do just that, and I explained to them what they had on their hands. In my opinion, it was a case of burking.

To *burke* means to murder by suffocation in a way that leaves few or no marks of violence. The name comes from an 1829 case in Edinburgh, Scotland, in which William Burke and William Hare were convicted of fifteen murders, after which they sold the bodies to the university's medical school to be used for anatomy classes. The bodies brought ten guineas each. Hare, the leader, turned against his partner and got out of prison in a few years. Burke, the follower, was hanged, and his body ended up on the very tables he had been filling. Their method of murder involved putting a hand over the nose and mouth of the intended victim while sitting on the victim's chest, thus preventing breathing. They did this thinking it left no marks.

But it can.

At dinner I explained that when I pointed out to Dr. Simms what I thought were petechial hemorrhages, he stated that he thought they were congested capillaries in the eye—that while blood had flowed into them, they had not, in fact, ruptured. This turned out to be an important distinction.

The prosecution had every reason to believe its own medical examiner. And, equally important, so might the jury. Outside experts can be perceived in many ways: hired guns, carpetbaggers, big-city big shots or, preferably, consummate professionals. But this was a rare situation: two expert witnesses—one hometown, one from New York—testifying for the prosecution that the manner of death was homicide, but disagreeing on the cause of death.

I told them that I knew this was not what they expected, that I knew the problems this could create and, if they wished, I could just go back to New York. But there was a legal problem.

If these had been defense attorneys I was meeting with, they would not have been compelled to reveal my findings to the prosecution. But, under the so-called *Brady* rule, established by the courts, the prosecution is compelled to reveal anything that might be helpful to the defense. But if the defense attorney finds anything harmful to his client, he cannot turn it over. His job is to defend the client. If he thinks the client is going to lie on the witness stand, he can ask the judge to be removed from the case, since he cannot participate in a lie, but he cannot turn over evidence that might indict or convict his client. He cannot destroy the evidence, but he can't point it out, either. The legal system is designed this way so that the defendants can give any and all information to their lawyers in protected confidence without fearing that their counsel will snitch.

For a defense attorney, winning is not solely a matter of getting a client acquitted. It is also about the degree of guilt, which is more subtle than simple guilt or innocence. Even if the defendant is guilty, he might not be guilty as charged. He might not be guilty of a capital offense, for instance, for which he could receive the death penalty, and the defense attorney is there to ensure that the verdict is not harsher than it should be.

The prosecutor's job, however, is to do justice. Sometimes that includes letting someone go. We are not supposed to prosecute people in this country just because we can make bad evidence fit the crime and the suspect. It is the prosecutor's job to find justice, and to do that, he must bring out all that he knows.

By my calling into question a portion of Simms's intended testimony, the defense could argue there was doubt on the accuracy of his findings—all of his findings. I was opening up the possibility that with this disagreement Simms and I could both be challenged by the defense counsel. We agreed on the manner of death as homicide but disagreed on the cause, and if the jury was confused by that concept, they might choose to disbelieve all of our other findings. It is hard to be perceived on the stand as a little bit wrong—wrong about one thing but not wrong about other things. And it appeared to me that Simms was wrong about the congested vessels in the eye and the source of the bruising on Binion's chest and around his mouth, and therefore about how Binion was killed.

But how would the jury react?

While I was sympathetic to the problems my opinion could create for the prosecutors, I was not about to change my medical determination. Under those circumstances, most prosecutors would have said, "Well, that isn't according to the evidence we have, so you must be wrong. Good-bye."

People frequently misunderstand this situation. When the public hears about these types of negotiations, they think there is some kind of intentional cover-up. But it isn't that. Experts can have different views.

Rogers and Wall made a bold decision. They chose to go forth and present both opinions in the preliminary hearing the next morning. Interestingly, between the time Dillard first called me and when I flew out to Las Vegas to review the records, I had been contacted by lawyers for the defendants to review their material. Had I been called by them first and looked at Simms's reports and photos, my opinion would have been the same. It's the independent science that guides my opinion.

When it comes to testifying, it is important for an expert witness to review in detail all of his findings and opinions with the attorney. This is called preparation. No expert should go into court without sufficient time to talk through the case with the attorney who calls him to the stand. In my opinion, the three most important factors in testimony are preparation, preparation and preparation.

Often, this does not happen. This is especially the case with medical examiners working for large cities. An autopsy performed today on a man hit by a city subway may not come to trial for five years, during which time the doctor has performed or overseen many other autopsies. Imagine—hundreds or thousands of autopsies later, the doctor is called by the city's counsel and told to be ready to testify without ever having discussed the matter. Tomorrow.

That is the worst case scenario, but at least there is a reason for it: Both sides are overworked. The infuriating cases, to me, are those where the attorneys just say to the expert witness, "Oh, you're the expert, you know what to do" or "You have testified in more murder trials than I have, so just do your stuff."

What that tells the expert is that the attorney does not understand the importance of preparation or does not want to spend the necessary time in preparing the case. Even something as mundane as explaining my qualifications, or how the lawyer will ask, "What is your occupation?" should be discussed ahead of time. Some experts like the attorney to say, "Tell us about yourself," and then let the expert speak at some length about his qualifications.

Handled poorly, this can sound a lot like the expert is bragging, and I learned early in my career by watching others not to allow anyone to put me on the stand and let me talk for a half hour about myself. It has made me feel very uncomfortable. Instead, I prefer to have it dragged out of me in the judicial process called qualifying. Whenever an expert testifies he has to be qualified—that is, the judge has to approve that the proffered expert is really an expert in the matter at hand.

Ideally, the attorney who calls me to the stand should follow a logical sequence of questions that leads me and, in turn, the jury, through five topics: my qualifications, the science I practice, the introduction and chain of custody of evidence, the examination and analysis of that material and, finally, my opinion.

There are twenty-four specialties in medicine. Within each specialty there are subspecialties. I am board certified, or a diplomate, in three subspecialties of pathology: anatomic pathology, which involves looking at the anatomy of the body and includes examining surgical specimens and performing autopsies; clinical pathology, which has to do with the chemistry of the body as tested in the laboratory; and forensic pathology, which has to do with investigation of unnatural and traumatic conditions that affect the body. All are more concerned with finding out why someone is sick or has died rather than with treating a patient.

The expertise of forensic pathology has long been accepted in the courts. But what about forensic climatology, forensic entomology, forensic botany? How about handwriting analysis, fingerprinting and blood-spatter analysis? All of these are currently being challenged as expert disciplines.

And what do we do with the lay expert? Movie buffs remember the scene in *My Cousin Vinny* in which the girlfriend testifies as a lay expert in auto mechanics. Should such a witness be allowed in court? She provided crucial testimony in the movie, but many judges would refuse to allow her onto the stand.

Evidence may be anything that the judge determines relevant

to a trial. It is important stuff and must be handled with great respect. Perhaps Herb MacDonell, the authority on blood spatter, says it best in his book *The Evidence Never Lies:*

> You can lead a jury to truth, but you can't make them believe it. Physical evidence cannot be intimidated. It does not forget. It doesn't get excited at the moment something is happening—like people do. It sits there and waits to be detected, preserved, evaluated, and explained. That is what physical evidence is all about. In the course of a trial, defense and prosecuting attorneys may lie, witnesses may lie and the defendant certainly may lie. Even judges may lie. Only evidence never lies.

Just because evidence exists, however, does not mean that it will find its way into court. In this country, we leave it up to the presiding judge to decide what the jury should hear, the so-called admissibility of evidence.

Beginning in the 1920s in America, scientific evidence was allowed into the courtroom if it was generally accepted by the scientific community. In 1993, however, the United States Supreme Court ruled in *Daubert v. Dow* that instead of "general acceptance," the new test of whether or not something was admissible in court could require an independent judicial assessment of the "reliability" of that evidence.

The old rule was called *Frye,* based on the 1920s case that established it. The new rule is called *Daubert,* and it applies in all federal cases and in those state jurisdictions that have adopted it as to deciding what will be heard as evidence in court. All courts make a determination of admissibility in either a pre-trial hearing or at trial, at which time the relevance of the material and the competence of the expert witness are judged. It can be grueling as well as confusing.

For instance, under *Daubert,* ballistics generally is acceptable as scientific evidence in the courtroom, while polygraphs are not. Under *Daubert,* cousin Vinny's girlfriend might not get in.

The language of the *Daubert* opinion gives broad discretion to trial judges and instructs them to consider at least four factors when determining admissibility: whether the theory or technique can be tested; whether the science has been offered for peer review; whether the rate of error is acceptable; and whether the method at issue enjoys widespread acceptance. Unfortunately, this is a huge burden on individual judges, who in general are not broadly educated in science.

Witnesses must be qualified in civil and criminal trials, preliminary hearings and grand juries, whether for the prosecution or the defense. I get up on the stand and am asked enough questions by the lawyer so that the judge can say, "Yes, you qualify to give expert opinions." This means that both my science and I can come to court. Then the judge will explain to the jury that the reason I have to be qualified is that from here on, I will be allowed, in this judge's courtroom, to give opinion testimony. Everyone other than the qualified experts will be giving fact testimony only: what they saw and when and where they saw it, not what they interpret it to mean.

The jury needs to know that the expert witness is in the courtroom to provide specialized information to assist it in interpreting the factual evidence. And the experts must be distinguished from fact witnesses.

Fact witnesses—the brother-in-law, the man on the street, the neighbor, the shop owner—come in and say, "I saw him." The expert witness comes in and says, "From my knowledge, experience, training and publications, I have found that you can't notice a reliable shape of the nose in this lighting condition." A fact witness who is a bank teller can say, "A woman came in, said, 'Give me a million dollars,' and then sat down and was twitching in her arms and her legs." An opinion witness who is a psychiatrist may say, "Based on my observations of her behavior, I can say that she was mentally ill at that time."

The forensic pathologist is usually both a fact and an expert witness—he both testifies to the facts of the autopsy findings and interprets their meaning. I may find that there are three gunshot wounds in the back. When I am called to testify about those facts, I am also usually asked to give an opinion about what the facts mean. The question will usually be "What is your opinion as to the cause of death?" The three bullet holes in the back are fact. Whether they are entrance or exit wounds is a matter of opinion. So in my testimony, I give a mixture of fact and opinion.

What the judge rarely mentions is something that attorneys love to bring out in court—who is paying whom and how much. Everybody loves to talk about the money expert witnesses make. There is an attitude that outside experts are hired guns because they get paid for their testimony, and the local medical examiner is trustworthy because he doesn't.

In general, medical examiners work for municipalities and are paid a salary to do the autopsy. Medical examiners are getting an annual salary, health benefits, job security, time to publish, academic advancement and promotions, which the outside expert does not get for his testimony.

Consider a civil litigation in which, for example, a person dies of multiple fractures. I can be called by the lawyer for one side and can certify the cause of death as multiple blunt force injury after being struck by a vehicle. That's all fact. He then may ask me, "How long did he live? How long was he conscious? How much pain and suffering did he endure? Could he have been saved if the ambulance had come sooner?"

When an expert is called into a criminal or civil matter for which he did not do the original fact work and for which he is not receiving a salary, he should be paid a fee. That's how our system of justice works. In the Binion case I was initially retained by the family to review what they thought was a murder but in which, after some time had passed, the local medical examiner had not yet made a determination. Subsequent to my involvement he did classify the death as a homicide, and the district attorney decided to retain me as a prosecution expert. It was an interesting twist, and one that some people found confusing.

It amazes me that, most of the time, juries are able to understand expert testimony. This, in part, is thanks to the judge, who explains to them that the reason experts are there is to help them gain insight and understanding into specialized knowledge that the average person does not have—whether it be anatomy, toxicology, forensic entomology or blood-spatter analysis. Expert witnesses are there to help them understand and interpret the evidence.

The preliminary hearing into the death of Lonnie Ted Binion went on to become one of the longest in the history of Clark County, Nevada. Nearly thirty witnesses testified over two weeks.

The hearing began on August 17, 1999. The next day, the local press recounted the proceedings at the hearing and recapped the death, stating that the death had been ruled a homicide and that "lethal quantities" of heroin and the prescription sedative Xanax had been found in Binion's system.

The burden of proof in a preliminary hearing is "slight or marginal evidence," far below "beyond a reasonable doubt," which is the degree of proof needed to secure a conviction at trial. Because of that, most defendants try not to bring out their best stuff at these hearings. They don't want to scoop their own experts whom they may need to call on at trial.

Doing what I always do on a day when I will be appearing as an expert witness in court, I dressed on August 19, 1999, in a dark suit and white shirt. My intention in this way of dressing is to show my respect for the jury.

Dr. Simms preceded me to the stand. As expected, he testified that the amount of heroin found in Binion's body was lower than what is normally considered to be lethal, but that the Xanax was far in excess of the fatal range. The autopsy report was reviewed. When David Rogers, the prosecutor, introduced the autopsy photographs, he dropped them on the defense table. Sandy Murphy, one of the two defendants, began to cry. She was allowed to leave the courtroom for five minutes to compose herself. Then she returned and heard, with everyone else, the findings of Dr. Simms. Cause of death: overdose. Manner of death: homicide.

I didn't see any of this—not in person or on television, which covered the entire proceeding—because while Dr. Simms was on the stand, I was inspecting Ted Binion's home, taking photos, looking at the place where the body had been found and generally getting a sense of the scene of the crime I believed had been committed.

Tom Dillard brought me to Binion's home, which was still sealed by the police. I was most struck by the odd way in which Binion had been found—on an exercise mat on a hard floor, where he had never previously slept, but which provided a good surface if someone wished to burke him. The mat was still lying on the floor. And it was also apparent to me from the curtains, which were open onto the garden, that the gardener would have been able to peer into the residence and see what was happening if the curtains had remained opened. The gardener testified that he noticed at the time of the death that the curtains were all drawn shut, which they had never been before. I was told that Binion's house was a big mansion, but it looked more like a large suburban ranch house with similar neighboring houses.

After lunch I was called to the stand. As always, I had with me my blue cloth carry-on bag. Inside were academic papers on the effects of chasing the dragon on the human body and on Xanax and heroin use, as well as copies of documents I had reviewed in the case. I took a quick look at the two young people sitting behind the defense table with their lawyers.

Sandy Murphy and Rick Tabish looked like a young couple in love. She was twenty-seven and he was thirty-four. They looked

very relaxed, casually small-talking. Tabish was married to someone else, with whom he had small children, and Murphy had lived
with Binion for three years. Although they might be facing the
death penalty for killing Binion, they looked very relaxed, almost
carefree. It was striking to me, accustomed as I am to seeing people sitting rigidly at the defense table.

At the time, Tabish was jailed but released for the preliminary
hearing. Murphy was under house arrest and was wearing an
ankle bracelet, which on one of the days of the hearing, she spray-
painted beige to match the miniskirted, formfitting suit she wore
to court.

When I testify at a trial, I always try to angle the witness chair
away from the defendants and more toward the jury than it is when
I get there. The expert witness is there to speak to the jury, after
all—not to the cameras in the courtroom, the gallery, the defendants, the lawyers or even the judge. Doing this is usually easier
during direct examination, when the lawyer I am working with will
cross over to the jury's side of the courtroom and allow me a clear
view of the members. During cross-examination, opposing counsel
will frequently try to train the expert's eyes off the jury. This is an
attempt to get the jury to believe you are ignoring them, that you
answer only to counsel. Later, when this case came to trial, the attorney would stand off to the right, forcing me to look away from
the jury—which I did, but only for the duration of the question, after which I would turn slightly and give my response to the jury.

There is great debate among attorneys over this practice. There
are those who think that juries in the twenty-first century don't
want eye contact with the witness, that they just want to view
everything as they do television: as disinterested observers, even of
their own lives. I don't buy this. My feeling is that it is better to
look at the jury and make eye contact. After all, they are the only
ones who matter once things get to court. I want to make contact
with them, to speak to them, to help explain the science I bring
with me to the courtroom.

How I speak is also an issue. I need to make things uncomplicated, and that's a fine line, because while I never want to talk down to a jury, I must bring the level of communication down to about a high school range, especially in science. And I must keep it interesting. Think for a moment about the weeks of DNA testimony in the O.J. Simpson case: After the trial many people said two things about it—that it was boring and that it was so complicated they didn't understand what was being said. This is less of a challenge in a preliminary hearing, since judges generally have more experience hearing scientific testimony, but even so, my testimony must be crystal clear.

The prosecution in the Binion case was bringing in not just one expert to testify to the cause and manner of death but two. And those two differed in their opinion. And with barely any time to prepare beforehand, I could not know just how the DA was going to handle this or whether the court would agree to amend the original criminal complaint charging Murphy and Tabish with murder to reflect my findings.

I also had no idea what reaction my findings would bring from the defense. They were well prepared, since the witness list and the expected testimony had been made public long before the hearing, with the exception of me and what I was going to say. I was almost a total surprise.

As the questioning began, I couldn't help but notice the amount of whispering Sandy Murphy did in her attorney's ear, her constant smiles and long glances over her shoulder at the gallery audience. Then came the review of the autopsy and the findings. I was asked what materials I had reviewed for the case: twenty-one tissue slides and more than two dozen Polaroid photographs. I stated for the record that I didn't accept drug overdose as the cause of death or agree that there was enough heroin or Xanax present to cause it. We examined and reviewed already introduced autopsy photos. I pointed out the bruises on Binion's lips, face and wrists, as well as those small, circular marks on the chest.

"What do those bruises suggest, Doctor?" asked Wall.

"The circular bruises are from shirt buttons."

It was then that I felt a change had taken place at the defense table. Murphy and Tabish had become rigid and were staring at me, their previous whisperings and light smiles gone. And in that instant, I had a feeling that I get only in courtrooms—the oddest sensation of a connection linking the defendant to the expert witness, when it seems that the defendant knows that someone else knows what happened. Murphy's and Tabish's dispositions appeared to me utterly changed. It would be fair to say that in the time it took for me to proceed through my testimony—stating for the record my expert opinion that Ted Binion had been hand-cuffed, laid on the mat on his back, and then smothered with a pillow or with someone's hands, that the cause of death was asphyxiation and that the manner of death was homicide—the blood seemed to drain from Sandy Murphy's face.

The preliminary hearing resulted in seventeen charges being brought against the lovers. They would be tried together for murder at a trial that began on March 27, 2000, and ended on May 19, 2000, when after eight days of deliberations, the jury came back with a verdict. It was never publicly revealed if there were odds on the trial, but this was Las Vegas, and you can pretty much bet that they favored acquittal.

But other numbers dominated the proceedings. We learned that Ted Binion had spent $1 million in his life on heroin. His drug dealer testified that Binion called him every three or four days to request three to four balloons of tar heroin, which the dealer would then deliver. On the day before Binion died, however, the drug dealer delivered twelve balloons, each containing a small amount of the tar heroin. We learned that in the weeks leading up to Binion's death, Murphy called Tabish sometimes thirty-one times in a single day on one of her three cell phones—but not once on the day the body was found. Murphy had originally arrived in Las Vegas only a few years before with her $20,000 life savings, which she promptly blew at the blackjack tables at Caesar's Palace, testimony revealed. That led her to work at Cheetahs, a topless club, where she modeled lingerie and where she met Binion, whose wife had just left him. On the first night he met Murphy, he offered her a wad of cash totaling $1,300, which she promptly threw back in his face, saying, "I don't want your money." She did not yet know that his net worth was somewhere between $35 million and $44 million.

Evidence included 386 marked exhibits for the prosecution, 167 for the defense, 2 prosecutors who questioned witnesses and 5 defense attorneys who did the same. The prosecution called 93 witnesses, the defense called 23.

I testified for the prosecution; Cyril Wecht, one of my closest friends and most admired colleagues, testified for the defense. This happens from time to time: Frequently, someone I know and respect will be on the opposing side. And that's just the way it should be.

As an expert, I would much rather have a proper forensic expert in my field, like Dr. Wecht, examining the evidence for the other side than a hospital pathologist not trained in unnatural death, as often happens.

Physicians may be the worst witnesses. They are often swayed by whoever asked them to be an expert. If that lawyer is smart enough to ask their advice, they conclude, he must know what he is doing. That being the case, physicians therefore adopt whatever the lawyer tells them as the facts of the case and become, if only subconsciously, an advocate for the lawyer rather than an independent adviser.

As a result of the preliminary hearing in the Binion case, the defense was compelled at trial to argue that Binion died of an overdose—either accidental or suicidal. Wecht had provided them with a seventeen-page report concluding that Binion died of "a combined heroin and Xanax overdose" as part of a planned suicide. He went on to write that he did "not find any evidence to support that contention that he was suffocated," and that he believed "Mr. Binion initially inhaled heroin smoke, as he had in the past, and this led to thoughts of suicide."

The defense attorneys did not share with Wecht all the information about the circumstances surrounding the death. Wecht and I did not look at the same set of facts, because we can look at only what is presented to us or what we request.

Part of the expert's obligation is to assume that he is not getting the whole story from the prosecutor or defense attorney. Everyone, after all, is biased and develops his or her own spin. The expert is not supposed to have innate prejudice, of course, but he is going to be influenced by what he looks at and must actively resist being biased toward either party.

In every trial it is the privilege of any attorney to search for what is known as "collateral material" on the experts, information that is not related to the issue of the trial but that will be used solely to attack the credibility of the expert. Prior testimony, for instance, is a fertile place for opposing counsel to go. What they choose to do with that information varies in each case. But we should always assume that they have it, ready to go if need be.

Dirt was flung in the Binion case. And the advance word on Court TV was that a defense expert and attorney named Jim Shellow had been flown in from Wisconsin just to cross-examine me. While I had never heard of him, much was made in the media about his skill and reputation in attacking medical experts.

He hammered away at me for four hours, emphasizing my differences with Simms and attacking my conclusions that the wrist bruises resulted from handcuffs. He suggested that the bruises might, instead, be from Binion's watchband. But I'm from New York City and have practiced forensic medicine for more than forty years, and I have seen a lot of handcuff abrasions—these were handcuff marks. After the trial someone who was not called as a witness told Tom Dillard that they were diamond-studded handcuffs purchased by Murphy in an expensive sex shop.

Shellow was a fine lawyer who trotted out most of the old standbys: He read to me from my own writings, lifting things out of context; he tried to anger me by suggesting I was biased; he implied that I was operating without the full range of facts (casting me as an out-of-towner, which I was); he differed with me when I referred to something as "the" official publication of the United States Department of Justice, and insisted instead that it was "an" official publication of the department.

If the expert lets stuff like that goad him, it's unfortunate, because the jury does not want to see a riled expert. They want to see a professorial, cool-headed, confident person who knows the science cold and has nothing in the past to be ashamed of.

Over and over it was suggested that I was under the thumb of what had become known at the trial as "The Binion Money Machine," that I was testifying to what the family wanted me to say. A lot was made of a statement I once made that I "enjoy" morgues. I do.

And for his part, when he gets on the stand, Wecht occasionally takes heat for appearing on a controversial 1995 television show, *Alien Autopsy: Fact or Fiction*. After forty years on the job, there's a lot of life to throw back at someone, which is why many attorneys opt for more inexperienced experts: no background, nothing to check.

Sometimes opposing counsel will revisit the high-profile cases I've worked on: everything from my work re-investigating the assassinations of John F. Kennedy and Martin Luther King, Jr., for Congress to my testimony in the O.J. Simpson case and my work in the Claus von Bulow murder trial, as well as my consultations in the deaths of the Romanov family and John Belushi.

Television is a great aid to those who want to embarrass the expert witness, as is the Internet. Sitting in the DA's office one afternoon on break, I was amazed to see the number of e-mails coming in to Wall from people watching the trial on Court TV, many of them suggesting that he undermine Wecht's testimony by asking him about the alien show.

These are called collateral attacks. And the information that is whizzing around on the Internet is feeding them faster than ever. Sometimes, of course, the exposure provides evidence, as it did in the Simpson case when someone outside the court sent in photographs of Simpson in Bruno Magli shoes, the likes of which produced footwear impression evidence in blood at the scene of the murder of Nicole Brown Simpson and Ron Goldman.

There is no way to know what really engages a jury—whom they believe and whom they dismiss. Experts are wrong to try to outguess juries. Experts are also wrong to think that their one day in court is so dramatic that it will determine the outcome of a trial.

The jury in the Binion case sat for all of April 2000 and into May. Then it deliberated for eight days. Finally, on Friday, May 19, just after 4 P.M., the jury reentered the courtroom of District Judge Joseph Bonaventure. Much was made by the media of the fact that four of the jurors were wearing sunglasses and that several appeared to be crying. It's questionable how true this is and what we should make of it, but no one could remember having ever seen such a sight in a jury.

Viewers at home watched on live TV as Sandy Murphy and Rick Tabish stood to learn their fate. The defendants remained standing as the foreman read seventeen separate guilty verdicts including that of murder. Appeals are pending.

I was not in court to see it. I didn't hear the news until two days later, when someone left me a message of congratulations. Those messages are hard to understand. To me there is no winning or losing at trial. An expert witness is too emotionally involved if he considers his testimony a win or a loss. It's my rule never to go to parties to celebrate what some think of as victories. I get invited, but I never go and didn't go to any for the Binion murder case. Even if I had wanted to, it would have been impossible for me to attend.

I was working.

Four

INSIDE

It is called the Y incision, but it is really more of a U
with a tail. Hand to glove, glove to scalpel, scalpel to skin—I've
done it twenty thousand times, and over the years the three-
pointed Y has morphed into a two-movement U.

The power of a scalpel is immense. Although light in the hand,
it pierces the skin with a tilt of the wrist. Years ago, I lost that hovering moment, waiting above the skin—the moment you see in
new doctors, that moment of hesitation. Now, I am eager to get in
and see what happened to the man who died during the holidays,
the man with the power cords wrapped around his neck found on
his living-room floor.

As soon as the scalpel plunges into the skin, you sweep it from
the left shoulder, down under the nipples and over to the right
shoulder: One motion, smooth and fast, and the skin parts like a
ravine. A small amount of blood passively leaks from the cut vessels, but since the heart is not pumping, there is no pressure

behind it. Then, lift the scalpel, place it at the bottom of the U and swoop to the pit of the abdomen, below the sternum, straight down, left of the belly button.

There are other types of incisions, but the Y is the most popular. It allows you to lift up and pull back the skin with ease. Also, it sews up well. You can go straight down from the chin, if you are looking for something along that line. And sometimes you are. If there is a question of subtle injury to the neck, as there is in manual strangulation, you cut straight down to more clearly visualize the windpipe, blood vessels and other structures of the neck and to see what injury, if any, is present.

Scalpel blades are very sharp, but they dull quickly when cutting through bone, cartilage and tissue. The blades are disposable and will be changed three or four times per autopsy to keep the edge. The handle remains; just pop off the blades. As with household knives, the sharper the blade, the more control you have and the less you cut yourself.

The national average is that pathologists cut themselves once in every seven autopsies. It's very easy to stick the scalpel into a finger, especially deep in the body when you are working blindly, mostly by touch, feeling for places to cut to release an organ into your other hand.

Most bodies don't have infectious agents, but of course some do, and you have to be careful. But the pathologists who wear metal mesh gloves—and many do, since the advent of the HIV virus—have lost the ability to feel their way through the body, the sense of knowing, simply by touch, that there is disease, swelling or a foreign object lodged in the organ at your fingertips. Some people call us cowboys, we pathologists who still wear only the latex gloves. They say it's macho. It's not. It's old school, plain and simple. And anyway, wearing the mesh gloves also makes small things difficult to pick up.

Picking up other things is one of the occupational hazards of forensic pathology. Mostly, just like babies, what we pick up are antibodies to everything around us, although over more than forty years, I've also picked up tuberculosis and hepatitis. In the 1960s, I cut my finger and developed a serious streptococcal infection called erysipelas, which caused the deaths of a number of autopsy pathologists in the 1920s and 1930s but was easily cured by penicillin when I became infected. However, during this treatment, I developed a huge butterfly rash on my face when it turned out I was allergic to penicillin. With the wonders of medicine come the side effects.

I lift my hands off the body at the end of the initial incision, there, left of the belly button, down at the pubic bone. Convention has us cut to the left of the navel because a ligament comes in from the right side, a remnant of the umbilical cord, but that same convention includes a respect for how we are born and forbids slicing that umbilical spot.

What had functioned perhaps just the day before as a closed system, a human life, is now laid open before the investigator, ready to be examined.

No one else has this privilege. And it is indeed a privilege to be the person allowed to search through this body for clues to the cause of death. Being the one person requested to do so by the family, or required to do so by the state, puts the medical examiner in a unique position as a doctor. We must respect that request: To find out everything that can be determined and then to speak up for the dead. And we must respect the process and the decedent. The body is sacred and entrusted to us, albeit very briefly.

How we decide who needs to be spoken for rests with the interests of society. Most people think that autopsies are automatic in cases of unnatural death. They're not.

The first decision at the scene of any death is made by the person finding the body, whether it is a nurse in the hospital, a family member sitting at the bedside or the police who have been called to a scene. In all deaths, someone needs to make some decisions, one of the first being who will sign the death certificate. That decision is governed by statutes that vary by state or county. Seventy-five percent of the time, a private treating physician issues the death certificate, and the death is not reported to the medical examiner's office. Of those cases reported to the medical examiner's or coroner's office, 75 percent result in the issuance of a death certificate after reviewing only the circumstances, the history and the body externally.

If a person has been treated for a life-threatening illness and is under the care of a physician, when death occurs that physician can issue the death certificate if he or she is of the opinion that the person died of that disease. Most people die in hospitals of natural causes, and for most of those deaths, no call is made to the medical examiner. An autopsy, in such a case, is performed by the hospital's pathologist only when the family requests it or gives permission.

In cases of suspicious or unnatural death, however, the body falls within the jurisdiction of the medical examiner or coroner, and an autopsy may be performed without the permission of the family because it has been determined that the needs of society outweigh the needs of the individual. In those cases, we don't put the family in the position to agree or disagree. In the case of the assassination of Martin Luther King, Jr., for instance, his widow was put under terrible pressure to agree to an autopsy. It was utterly unnecessary: It was a murder; an autopsy should be done.

When I come down to the autopsy room, I have to make a decision whether or not the body presents enough problems and whether there are enough circumstances surrounding the death to require me to do an autopsy. Sometimes I say no, it looks like a natural death, only to find that the wishes of the family are that one be done. Although any taxpayer has a right to request an autopsy, the financial burden may fall on the family, and that stops a lot of people from requesting one. In this way, death investigation favors the rich: Families who can afford it can hire private pathologists. And many do. I disagree with this system and think that if it falls within my jurisdiction and the family requests one, an autopsy should be performed without charge.

The result is that most suicides are not autopsied. Neither are most fatalities in auto accidents, despite the fact that an autopsy can provide a lot of information about how that person died and how to develop better safety features. If someone is shot in the head and lies in a coma for years and then dies, an autopsy should be done, since an assault has now become a murder and someone may need to stand trial.

Every case is different, and every case deserves the most professional attention available, which is another problem. In my role as a witness for the dead, I speak for those whose deaths we question. I have tried to speak for those as diverse as Martin Luther King, Jr., John F. Kennedy and the nine dead infants of an upstate New York woman named Mary Beth Tinning. I have testified more than a thousand times. First I perform pathology, then I engage in forensics: I examine, then I give public testimony. That is what forensic pathology is.

It's a long tradition. After examining the body of Julius Caesar, the physician Antistius spoke to the senators assembled in the Forum, reporting that there were twenty-three stab wounds in the fallen leader, but only one was fatal. However, it is not ancient Rome, but the England of the Middle Ages that provided the model for modern American medical death investigation, and that is one reason so many unnatural deaths today remain a mystery.

In the eleventh century, the king of England, needing to maintain the size of his army, decided to tax any intentional loss of life. If someone in your family committed suicide, his property was forfeited to the monarchy. If you killed someone with your horse and cart, the animal and vehicle were absorbed by the crown. Of course, people tried to avoid the tax, even to the point of covering up suicides. So in 1194, King John, spurred by the ransom demand for his brother, Richard I, captured during the Crusades, established an office to collect the debts he thought the crown was owed. Those who enforced the law were called *crowners*. They were tax collectors, untrained in determining the cause of death.

By the 1700s, the job, its title corrupted to *coroner,* had been exported to America. Of all the traditions we inherited from England, this, regrettably, is among the least changed.

Today, half of all American counties employ a coroner to investigate unnatural death. Most coroners are untrained in medicine. Frequently they are undertakers, but they are also plumbers, bookkeepers and, only occasionally, doctors. But they are always politicians, for coroner is an elected position. There are but two qualifications in most jurisdictions: You must be a citizen of the United States and you must be over twenty-one.

The other half of our counties employ medical examiners for this work. All of them are physicians. But fewer than four hundred are full-time forensic pathologists—physicians with extra training in determining the circumstances of death and explaining them in a legal forum.

We also lack national standards for investigating unnatural—homicide, suicide and accidental—deaths and for protecting, documenting and collecting evidence at the crime scene. In some communities, police follow strict rules at the scene to preserve and collect evidence. In most communities, however, the standards are much more lax.

In other words, we lack a uniform method for examining unnatural death. We don't do right by the dead.

Our most tragic example of this occurred on November 22, 1963. The body of President John F. Kennedy was examined by hospital physicians in Dallas. After the body was returned to Washington, hospital pathologists who had no training or experience in gunshot wounds performed an examination. It would have saved this nation years of heartbreaking speculation if a forensic pathologist with homicide experience had performed the autopsy. It might have hushed the conspiracy rumors that had already begun to spread.

Medical examiners are rarely needed to establish the cause of violent death. Usually the bullet wounds, the strangulation marks, the stab wounds speak all too well for themselves. But proper medical examination can dispel the questions that hover around unnatural death.

That could have been done even in 1963. Now, it should be a matter of course.

Where solving a crime once hinged on confessions, eyewitnesses and that time-honored tradition of the snitch, we can now depend on science—but only if that science is utilized by trained and experienced professionals in every precinct and every county. Without it, murders—even those whose trials run for months on national television—go unsolved.

In fact, the very people who are supposed to protect and defend frequently go into court lacking the evidence they need to determine guilt or innocence in even the most heinous crime. That evidence can be as subtle as a fiber or as obvious as a bloody print made by the sole of an Italian shoe. But it's always there. And frequently it is literally stepped on—or over—by people at the scene. Sometimes the evidence drips away in blood when someone flips over a body to take it to the morgue.

Of course, pathology without policy won't do. Colorado has so few homicides that the police who responded first to the JonBenet Ramsey crime scene in Boulder did not adequately protect the scene, and as a result, valuable evidence may have been lost, leaving everyone to second-guess what should have been done in the first critical hours at that crime scene.

Every body that is presented to a coroner, medical examiner or attending physician will be accompanied by some set of facts. These facts can range from a full medical and family history including time, manner and cause of death, to the slimmest of details. Capable people should be making the decisions of when to investigate. But that is not always the case.

At each autopsy I am very much aware in my own mind that

every gut is different, that every person is different and that I am going into a temple. I am constantly aware, as usual as it is for me to do this procedure, that for this individual, this is the only time an autopsy will be done. Everyone leads a unique life, and at autopsy the findings reflect that. I, as the pathologist, am suddenly the only person given permission to look, to give this type of internal exam that no one—no surgeon, no matter how extensive the procedure—has ever done on this person's body. And I am doing it as a legal requirement, which may be against the wishes of the family. But we have to do it. The needs of society to know and to document what happened in a way that can then be presented in a courtroom outweigh the wishes of the family. Otherwise, the person responsible for the death might not be punished.

So I had better get it right the first time. After that, the Sanctity of the Sepulchre takes hold. It's common law that shifts the balance of power away from the state almost as soon as I am done. Before the body is buried, the state can do many things. After the body is in the ground, however, the family has more control and gets to decide whether I am allowed to look. So you want to look thoroughly and with great respect for the mission of answering for the dead. You don't want to rush and you don't want to miss anything, because you might never again be invited back. And what's more, despite how obvious the cause of death might seem, we have a responsibility to do a full and complete autopsy. That means I am going to look at everything.

The man on the table today deserves it, after all. Someone killed him, and justice must be served. At my elbow are the items that will assist my hands to get into his body to have a look: the scalpel, with its slender blade; an electric vibrating saw, to open up the skull cavity and cut through the ribs (or clippers, which also do the latter); a little twisting device, like a screwdriver, that separates the top of the skull where the saw has cut through; a bread knife, to section the liver and the brain; two kinds of scissors, one with a sharp edge for opening small parts of the body and the other, a blunt-edged pair for the intestinal tract; and the most important instruments of all—the ruler and the scale.

A lot of organ description is subjective; people see colors differently and assess rigidity based on their individual sense of touch. But there are standard ranges against which to measure the weight and size of organs. One pound is the equivalent of 454 grams. A normal heart runs from 320 to 350 grams in weight; more than 400 grams is considered enlarged. So it's a small organ, despite the fact that our lives depend on it. The biggest organ in the body is the liver, weighing between 1,200 and 1,500 grams, or about three pounds.

Animals all have essentially the same organs and skeletal structure: A giraffe has the same number of neck and spine bones as a human; a mouse has a heart, liver, lungs, kidneys and gallbladder. Even a nonmammalian, one-celled paramecium can do all the things we do with billions of cells: It breathes, eats, defecates and moves. Plants use food, use up carbon dioxide and give up oxygen. Looking at the array of life on this planet makes one appreciate the wonder of what's inside.

Humans are wonderful, with so many special functions in our organs that have developed over billions of years. A kidney by itself is a miracle. But what always amazes me is the intricate connections of the human body.

After the incision, the skin is pulled, or reflected, back, and you can immediately note the color of the tissues. In cases of carbon monoxide poisoning, for instance, the muscles will be pinker than in other bodies, because the carbon monoxide molecule combines with iron in the hemoglobin molecule in the red blood cells to produce a bright pink color. The thickness of abdominal wall, called the panniculus, composed mostly of fat (called adipose tissue) in the abdomen, tells you the state of nutrition of the person. One to two centimeters is normal. Three is considered fat.

The models in women's fashion magazines amaze me: All of them would be considered emaciated by any forensic pathologist. And they would be listed as such on an autopsy report. Normal bodies have a layer of fat.

Using the scalpel and cutting under the tissues, I pay close attention when dissecting between the skin and the rib cage. The skin is very thin at that point, and I don't want to cut through and "buttonhole" or inadvertently cut from below and make a hole in the outer skin, which would cause problems in the embalming process. I also don't want to cause inadvertent fractures of the ribs themselves. The abdominal musculature is thin, and most of the abdominal wall consists of an average of an inch thickness of yellow fat.

The drama of the ribs is how they thrust upward, harboring the heart and lungs. But they must be penetrated. What connects the ribs to the sternum, the necktie-shaped bone running down the chest, is merely costal cartilage that can be easily cut through. Underneath the sternum are the left and right internal mammary arteries, which in recent years have become important in coronary artery surgery. The individual bands of cartilage are cut with a scalpel, clippers or a saw. It's a personal choice which tool to use but also a practical one, depending on the age of the deceased. If the person is less than thirty years old, the cartilage in front is easily cut through with a sharp knife. Older, and it is calcified and harder. Your ear, for instance, is made of cartilage. It is hard but pliable. As anyone who has ever tried to pierce one soon discovers, it does not give up easily to a needle but requires a certain energy to enter. So it is with the rib cartilage.

The man whose body we have here is more than fifty years old. I need a new blade as soon as I've cut through the ribs.

Laying aside the sternum and its connected cartilage, I see that the moist insides of the body shine with their distinctive colors. And immediately the uniqueness of the body before me reveals itself. Since we die as we live, habits both good and bad are laid out under the eyes of the examiners.

First there are the anatomical quirks. Everyone has them: A hiatal hernia may crimp the stomach and form a pouch above the diaphragm; an enlarged heart gone undetected shows itself for the first time; smokers' tarred lungs look ghastly. The left testis normally is lower than the right. If the right one is lower, it is a sign that inside the body the organs are reversed. This is called *situs inversus*, meaning that the organs are transposed. The heart will be on the right side of the chest, instead of the left; the liver will be on the left side of the abdomen, not on the right.

And so, in every autopsy there will be something unique, something never seen before, and something to learn. Inside stomachs I've seen ears that were bitten off in fights, and worse. Once, a man cut off his own penis and swallowed it, bleeding to death in the suicide. Why didn't it hurt to cut himself that way? Because bleeding to death is not painful to someone who is emotionally ill, which is why pepper spray doesn't work on emotionally deranged people: They don't feel it. People will report that someone in a struggle fought on and on despite a beating and will assume that the person had super strength. It's not true. Emotionally disturbed people aren't any stronger, they just don't react to pain in the same way, and so they struggle longer. The results can be seen at autopsy, and if the mental history is available and you do a thorough job, you learn. And then you teach. These are things the police need to know.

Every time we open a body we are private witnesses to all the things done to it: alcohol consumed, sexual habits pursued, children born or the reasons no pregnancy came to term. Exercise habits show up in the musculature and bone density. Drug use, family problems, line of work and domestic violence—we compare what we see against what is normal and note it all.

Most deaths that end up under the jurisdiction of the medical examiner turn out to have been natural. The person just died unattended, and so we have to investigate.

The organs are first examined in situ, or in place, in their normal relationships to one another. Then, they come out by one of two methods, both named for German pathologists. Using the Rokitansky procedure, they all come out at once. This is how interns and residents do it, mostly because it is easier for their supervisors. With the Virchow method, each organ is removed separately and immediately examined.

It's 3:15 P.M. in this autopsy, and while I personally prefer not to turn on the air conditioning—it can blow bugs around as well as blow trace evidence away—I agree to allow it back on. As soon as it starts to cool and refresh the autopsy suite, everyone looks visibly relieved. I frequently forget that people really are bothered by the dead air.

After cutting open the pericardial sac around the heart, I will observe whether there is any blood accumulated there. Injuries sustained from hitting a steering wheel or the back of the seat in front of you, for instance, can cause a buildup of blood in this area, which will, in turn, prevent the heart from fully expanding and doing its job. This is what killed Princess Diana, who, by not wearing a seat belt, left herself open to the massive fatal injuries to her chest. It is interesting to note that in France emergency medicine is performed on site—in her case, by the side of the road. This is great medicine for heart attacks because it saves people. But in the United States the practice is to scoop and get to the hospital, which would have allowed Diana to undergo immediate surgery to relieve the bleeding. That may well have saved her life.

Before I remove the heart, I stick a needle and syringe in it and collect blood. I also collect a urine sample from the bladder. I send both off to the lab for a toxicology check. Later I will take a sample of the stomach contents. If there is a gunshot wound to the heart, blood can be taken from another site. The brain can be used for alcohol detection, for instance, since it is in a protected area of the body.

Other fluids that may be collected include those in the eye. If a body has bled out, it may be necessary to test this fluid for drugs and for electrolytes, which can be very helpful in judging time of death since potassium in eye fluid rises in a predictable level after death.

Then the heart is removed by cutting through its attachment to the veins and arteries that enter and leave its four chambers. This takes about thirty seconds. When you are holding a heart in your hand, it is impossible not to marvel at the work of this machine. It pumps five to six quarts of blood every minute over sixty thousand miles of blood vessels to reach all the tissues of the body. It beats all the time, whether you're awake or asleep; it will do so two to three billion times by the time you reach your eightieth birthday.

I place the heart on the stainless steel tray and dissect it open with a knife and scissors, following the route of the flow of blood: right atrium, right ventricle, left atrium, left ventricle. The arteries are either then crosscut, like slicing a bread loaf, or cut through with tiny scissors in a long, continuous slice. Long ago, after I had done this only a few times, I realized how unequal everybody is: Some people are born with large arteries, giving them an advantage in longevity over those with narrow ones, which are more easily obstructed by plaques. Interestingly, this has no correlation to stature. I know of no study that has ever examined the arteries of generations of the same family to see if size is hereditary and, if so, whether it follows maternal or paternal lines or is the result of pure chance as many other things are.

After serially transecting the coronary arteries, I look inside. And here it is: The widow maker, the beginning of the left anterior descending coronary artery, where heart attacks usually start. The hemodynamics caused by the turbulence of the blood here usually makes this area the first to clog. Half a centimeter down, this man's left anterior descending coronary artery is 80 percent blocked. That would have qualified him for bypass. And anyone with that much blockage will die more quickly of neck compression than someone with clear arteries. I have to tell them, the prosecutors and cops standing here—they hate to hear it—and they have to tell the defense. And the defense attorneys will pick up on this, if they are smart. Or they might skip right over it. A man with this much blockage, engaging in rough sex—say, sex that included a little strangulation, thought to heighten the orgasm—will die faster than someone without this kind of blockage.

This is severe coronary arteriosclerosis. Most strangulations are intentional, but a good defense attorney might even say that in today's case, all the defendant meant to do was knock the guy out and get out of there, and he staged it by placing the cords around the dead man's neck for some reason or another. If the defense attorney isn't good, the assailant could very well end up facing capital punishment. But a good lawyer might argue that it was consensual rough sex, that nobody was supposed to die, that his client got scared and ran. That's a whole lot different in intent—and in jail time—than setting out to murder someone by strangulation and steal his car.

"Car's been found, Doc. We got it."

Some things have simply disappeared from autopsies. For instance, syphilitic aortitis and rheumatic heart disease, which have been largely banished with the widespread use of penicillin. That miracle of mold greatly reduced the number of streptococcal infections. They used to say that strep throat infections licked the joints and bit the heart because they caused joint pain and, in about 3 percent of the cases, developed into rheumatic heart disease. Not much anymore in the United States.

The lungs are removed, one at a time. The right lung, with three lobes, is larger than the left lung, which has two. The heart, which is on the left side of the chest, takes up that extra space. The lungs must be checked to see if they are well aerated and also for color.

This man didn't smoke, but the lungs are congested, which corresponds with the coronary blockage. The right lung weighs 680 grams, the left one 510. I can tell he didn't smoke because smokers, like coal miners, have a black pigment in their lungs. Lungs should be pink. We can tell in an instant if the person was a city or country dweller. People from Puerto Rico, for instance, who die soon after moving to New York City have very pink lungs. The longer they stay, the less pink they will be. People who leave the city keep their tarnished lungs, though, since soot, like carcinogens, tends to hang around.

All of the organs are sectioned, and from those sections are taken tiny samples for microscopic testing. Under the microscope we look for diseases such as hepatitis or small cancers that can't be identified by the naked eye. Going through the body methodically, we look at the weight and condition of each organ and then describe each one in terms of its architecture and color: the yellow fatty enlargement of the liver from alcoholism; the scarring of the spleen by sickle-cell anemia; the granularity of the kidneys in high blood pressure.

The man on the table this morning was last seen in public while eating in a bar. There is a record of what he ate and the witnesses to it, including the waitress on duty that night. The man was not alone. But this was days ago—perhaps as long as a week. Will the food still be in his stomach? And will it be what he ordered, or did he live long after the meal and perhaps eat something else before he died? There is only one way to find out.

"We know what he had for dinner?"

The detective looks at his notes.

The stomach looks like a small, saggy pink pouch when removed. It slits open with the touch of a scalpel. The contents are scooped out with a stainless steel ladle and spread out for a look. Some of it will go to the lab for analysis. Since 90 percent of what we eat moves out of the stomach in two to three hours, we can tell how long before he died the food was consumed. Sometimes we can even tell where the person ate, or we can match the meal to eyewitness accounts of when he was last seen. In this case, though, the food is all gone. We now know it was more than a few hours between his last meal and when he was killed.

The appendix, which no longer functions in our bodies, can be a great stumbling point for many medical examiners. It sits there, a small, fingerlike appendage sticking out at the beginning of the large intestine, unnoticed and unremarkable. Miss it, though, and it will come back to haunt you. Defense attorneys like nothing more than to ask a medical examiner on the stand, "And what was the condition of the appendix?" "Unremarkable" is the typical answer. And you had better hope it was, because if, in fact, that appendix was removed from the dead man when he was twelve, the jury may not believe anything you say from that moment on. So, we note its presence or absence for the record by stating, "Appendix: Normal," on the autopsy report, even if it is not a cause of death. It's a dead giveaway of a shoddy autopsy otherwise.

Testes shrivel with age. In women, we check the state of the cervix and the uterus, noting the phase of menstruation. Suicide occurs more often during menstruation than otherwise. People like to ask if it's true that homicide is more common during PMS, but I wouldn't know: We don't get the murderer in the morgue; we get the victim. Things check and balance in the body—at least they should. A woman who is still menstruating is unlikely to have any visible symptoms of heart disease because estrogen protects against it. The body is an astonishing system.

The point of deadly contact between the deceased and his assailant is believed to be the neck. That is where the power cords were found, looped around his throat. Cutting inside the neck to remove the larynx, hyoid bone and thyroid cartilage is dangerous because you can't see and you can easily run into your own scalpel. This is where most pathologists typically cut themselves. After removing the hyoid bone, I lay it out next to the body. It appears to be intact. Not so the left greater cornu of the thyroid cartilage: It is fractured at its juncture with the ala, or body of the cartilage. *Thyroid,* from the Greek, means "shield-shaped." The right thyroid cartilage is fractured at its distal third. All show focal areas of surrounding hemorrhage. This was a traumatic asphyxia strangulation of the neck, no doubt about it.

"Got it. Strangled. Want to see?"

In the course of the last half hour, the room has filled up. Looking up, I count twelve people, including Wayne, the diener, and me. The detectives on the job are here, and their supervisors have come in. Some of the cops who were working the scene have come over to compare notes. The prosecutor on the job is here. Everyone has milled around for ten minutes or so, talking; some have questions, others eat donuts or drink soda. Some brought in their own cups of coffee. One guy is wearing full camouflage gear, including huge black boots that lace up over his pant legs. He and his partner, in jeans, are working undercover. A couple of the guys have been in and out for smokes. They don't seem in much of a hurry, walking around the body, asking questions and catching up on what we know by now.

"You grabbed some trace, I understand?" a man in a trench coat asks the two undercover cops.

The guy in the boots nods.

"You gonna fingerprint him, right?" asks another, pointing his chin at the portable kit for doing just that.

The detectives who stay for the entire procedure don't, as a rule, suit up. But they can. One of the detectives did today and is wearing gloves and a plastic apron.

"Hey, Dave, you look like you're ready for lobster," someone says to him.

A beeper goes off. Everyone goes for his or her belt.

Talking to them, I pick up the scalpel and walk to the head of the dead man. Once there, I press the blade into the scalp and circumnavigate the skull. This is the second incision to the body. The Y-shaped incision—despite the fact that it is not one continuous cut—is considered the first. The scalp incision, ear-to-ear behind the head, is the second. After it is cut, the scalp is then folded so that it will sit like a tight cap over the dead man's closed eyes.

The ADA visibly relaxes. Until now, he's been standing behind a chair in the little area nearer the coolers than the body.

"This is better," he says, removing his jacket. "It's like he isn't watching us anymore."

Then Wayne picks up the circular saw, and it seems as though everybody has somewhere else to be. The brain makes people very uncomfortable, especially when you're about to take it out of the head. The three men in trench coats look at their watches, in sync, then at one another, and they're out of there. The plainclothesmen are next, and within the ninety seconds it takes to get that saw up and moving, we are back to just Wayne, two detectives, the ADA and me. Nothing clears a room like removing a brain.

As it moves once around the skull, the saw casts off fine white dust in all directions. Then Wayne puts down the saw and inserts a small chisel-like device, which he twists to pop open the skull. He then removes the skullcap.

The dura around the brain is the first thing you see. It is the thick, protective membrane covering the brain, and it immediately tells us about the functioning of the individual. A blood clot above it (epidural) or below it (subdural) indicates that the person has suffered a severe traumatic injury. After removing the dura, one can readily see the sulci, which are the spaces between the gyri, or ribbonlike wrinkles of the brain. These differ only slightly from individual to individual; the brain of a genius at autopsy looks like the brain of a schizophrenic. With injury, tumors or meningitis, the brain swells and the gyri and sulci become flattened. The wrinkles of the brain become more prominent with age, as brain cells die; the brain, which normally weighs 1,200 to 1,300 grams, can easily weigh less than 1,100 grams before death. As the brain cells diminish, the normal ventricular system running through the brain expands.

Damage from any blows to the top of the brain will be evident now. Bruises take a long time to heal; even with a balding man, like the one before us, bruises not immediately visible on the scalp may appear on the ribboned surfaces of the brain.

There is some bruising to the brain here. The detectives check their notes. There was no visible damage to the coffee table in the dead man's living room. No sign that he hit his head on it. But they get on the walkie-talkie anyway and ask their peers at the murder scene to check it out again.

The brain is gently removed by cutting through the juncture between the lower medulla and the spinal cord and I lay it on the corkboard on the autopsy table.

"It's getting mushy," Wayne says.

Decomposition will do that. Wayne goes back to the head, where he wipes out the empty cranial cavity.

Slicing the brain with the bread knife, I am looking for any abnormalities. Head injury victims actually die from swelling of the brain after the blow, as the brain expands and pushes down on the brain stem, where the control mechanisms for breathing and heart function are located.

Although there are no abnormalities I can see with the naked eye, I still cut a small sample with the scalpel to look at under the microscope.

In this case, this day, things move quickly. But not always. If there had been a gunshot, for instance, I would have to follow the bullet's path through the body and retrieve it and all of its fragments. In some cases legs and arms are dissected. But that is not necessary here.

It's not that you autopsy just to get what you need. You get more than what you need, but there are some things you just don't need to do. In cases where we know very little about the dead, more extreme measures may be necessary. But always, we try to do only what is needed.

If a long-buried body turns up in the morgue, we may need the expertise of a forensic odontologist, who will examine the jaws and study the teeth and dental work. In some cases, facial reconstruction may be the only way to determine identity and the skull will be sent to an expert, whose painstaking job it is to rebuild a face using clay, sketches and computer imaging.

I have heard of hands being cut off at autopsy and sent to fingerprint experts, but almost always that is unnecessary. Any good fingerprint person knows that if a body has dried out, all you have to do is inject saline under the skin to bring out the ridges.

Only once in more than forty years have I had to remove a hand. It was the Sacco case in the late 1980s. Earlier, when police were investigating an organized crime case, the defendant tried to make a deal by telling the investigators that he knew where a body was buried in a big industrial landfill in Orange County, New York. The police excavated the site but found nothing. Then a year or two later, when another suspect told them the same story, the detective on the case figured there must be something at this site. Another dig was arranged, this time involving the Orange County Police, the New York State Police, the FBI, the New Jersey State Police (the murder of the man whose body they were looking for allegedly occurred in New Jersey) and the New York State attorney general.

For five days, big cranes pulled up all kinds of metal from the industrial site. On the fifth day, up came a body from the dumpster. I quickly went to the scene, since I didn't want it moved unnecessarily. The body had on the clothes the witness said the victim was wearing when he was shot. It was the right height and weight. We brought the body back to the Orange County morgue. The man had been missing for two years, so there was a lot of decomposition. We took dental X rays to compare them to those of the man who was missing.

Dr. Lowell Levine, a great forensic odontologist, looked at the X rays and gave us a startling answer: It was the wrong guy. The teeth didn't match the missing man's dental records. Now the fingerprints became very important.

Looking at the hand, I didn't see much in term of prints. The New York State Police senior investigator on the case, Ralph Gagliardi, agreed. After two years in the ground, of course, you can't expect much. So the FBI offered to try to lift the prints if

Gagliardi took the hands to the FBI lab in Quantico, Virginia. Keeping the hands moist, Gagliardi flew them down by New York State Police jet. The lab technicians worked on rehydrating them and got one usable print with enough ridges and details off an index finger. It was him, all right, the guy we had been told it was.

But what about those teeth? We never learned if the X rays were innocently mislaid or deliberately planted.

So taking off a hand is rare. In some decomposed bodies, the outermost layer of skin on the hand will deglove—literally come off—and you just need to put your own gloved finger into it and roll off a print or two. But I never fingerprint at the beginning of an autopsy since to do so would destroy trace evidence. I wait until the end.

You do what you need to do because that is what the dead deserve. But you don't do more than necessary because they deserve that as well.

The deceased also deserve privacy, and it's up to me to ensure that. All through the autopsy the detectives and I take pictures to document what we do as well as to allow the experts on the other side (in this case, the defense) to review the work done in the morgue. Photographs are tricky business these days—good, brisk business in the wrong hands. The autopsy photos of the famous sometimes end up in the tabloids, just where you don't want to see them. So you have to be careful—both in who takes them and where you get them developed.

Normally the places I take my film to be developed know the kind of work I do. But the one-hour developing places that have emerged over the last twenty years are a dream come true for me. I can sit and wait for the results, especially in such cases as O.J. Simpson's. I photographed Mr. Simpson as I examined him to document any injuries and to collect hair specimens. As it turned out, only minutes later he slipped out and fled in the white Bronco in the famous highway chase. Those photos are not the kind I want sitting at a developer for days. I waited as the film was developed.

Of course, mistakes have been made. Photos taken of John Lennon by a mortuary person after Lennon's murder made it onto the cover of the *New York Post*. And JFK's autopsy photos are available on the Web, as are those of many other celebrities. It's a shame. This is not a procedure that should be viewed by anyone other than those who need to know the details in pursuit of truth.

Autopsy photos always include something to judge the scale of what is being shot. Kodak makes the traditional, six-inch autopsy ruler, which is 18 percent gray and allows the developer to know how to process the film for color accuracy.

The other record is the autopsy report, transcribed and typed up from the notes I make into my tape recorder. I wait until the end of the exam to record my findings. Unlike some medical examiners, I don't say much during the dissection, weighing and observing. Things are sometimes not what they first appear to be: What at first may look like an entrance wound may, in fact, turn out to be an exit wound. An incorrect first impression, recorded on tape, may come back to haunt me at trial.

When I started out in the 1960s in New York City, I worked in a brand-new building. It was state of the art at the time. Of course, it included the latest dictation equipment so that every table—there were eight—had a microphone hanging over it. Underneath the table was a foot pedal that started and stopped the Dictaphone belt. You could dictate as you went along. And for a while this seemed like a really good idea. A whole generation of buildings followed, equipped with the mikes hanging over the tables.

The problem soon emerged. Those microphones quickly got clogged up with the blood and tissue that are plentiful in an autopsy room. They were soon taken away. Many places use a blackboard, so the medical examiner can have someone jot down weights and notes without the medical examiner having to take off his gloves. I don't like that. I like to take off my gloves and think about what I might be missing, walk around the body and imagine myself in court, wondering what I might need to know then.

I dictate twice: after the external exam and then again after the internal. As I am performing the internal examination, I call out the weights and measurements to a cop, who jots them down on a mimeographed sheet I give out. Other than that, I keep my findings to myself until I talk into the handheld recorder as I walk around the open body at the end of the autopsy. That way I can dictate the complete trajectory of a bullet, the total damage of a slashing, the entire crime scene that is a body.

The dictation of my findings becomes the autopsy report, one of about a dozen documents that a medical examiner's office may generate on every case. Others include the notice of death, which records when the case was first called in, and the death certificate. My tape recordings officially become an autopsy report after they are transcribed. In a medical examiner's office, there are secretaries who do this work. When I was the New York City medical examiner, we had such a high volume of autopsies—seven to eight per day—that there were people whose jobs were dedicated solely to transcription. These days I have a private transcriptionist who has learned the jargon. It's a very specific language, the language of the morgue.

At the end of the autopsy, Wayne will return the organs to the body cavity. The important specimens—in this case, the fractured thyroid cartilage—will be saved in a jar as evidence. They will join the jars lining the walls of this room, all the tissue awaiting its day in court. It's a tiny room, getting smaller with every autopsy. Jars of tissue are packed in tight among rows of slide boxes, on which there are more tissue samples. In this particular room, there is a box of breast implants that have been removed, dated and stored for possible civil action.

Wayne is working slowly, tired after his second autopsy of the day. He looks exhausted; even the tattoo on his upper right arm is barely flexing.

"Two today, huh?"

"Hey, you pick your victims as you find 'em," says Wayne, shrugging.

He will finish packing the body, including the brain, and then sew up the incisions with the large, looping movements of the baseball stitch.

A week later an autopsy report is delivered to those who need it. It is five pages long. Page one states the name, birth date, date of discovery and autopsy date of the dead man. At the bottom it says:

> Cause of death: Asphyxia by compression of neck
> Manner of death: Homicide

Five

HENRY

Rarely will he have a driver, since Dr. Henry C. Lee prefers to be out on his own in his Dodge Intrepid, cleaving the traffic on Connecticut's highways. Now going eighty miles per hour, the man in the black suit and black shoes grips the black cell phone in one hand and the black steering wheel in the other and whisks the black car past everything else on the road. The only measurable evidence of the arcing velocity is the silent, lighted speedometer, which is as steady as Lee himself, a man obstinately unshaken by the pace. The pristine vehicle smells like a brand-new car, hinting to a terrified passenger that this just might be a body shop's loaner to a good and constant customer.

As he drives, Dr. Lee looks like a man who has nothing to fear, which is odd, since he works in a world of murder, mayhem, blood spatter, the press, chaotic crime scenes, ceaselessly ringing phones, vibrating beepers, incessant pleas from desperate next of kin, calls from Congress and nationally televised testimony in high-profile murders, not to mention that matter of a blue wool Gap dress and the DNA samples taken from a president of the United States. He drives as he does because he is never stopped by a cop unless it's for his autograph.

But he looks like a man in nothing so much as what one side of dogma calls a state of grace and which the flip side might refer to as a perpetual state of charm. And while they'd both be a little bit right, any good marketing person would recognize in an instant that here is the rarest of all American dreams—the perfect mix of medium and message in one man.

Everybody always talks about Henry Lee in terms of how much he works—long hours, long days—but that is too simple an observation when gathering the evidence on him. You also have to factor in the speed at which he travels in order to sum up how one living man can be a national hero simultaneously in Taiwan and mainland China and also be literally beloved on both sides of justice, from one end of America to the other. It can't be just the long hours, despite the fact that every newspaper and magazine profile of him will note that Henry is impossible to shadow, that he lives an eighteen-hours-a-day, seven-days-a-workweek life and that television producers compare tales of securing permission to follow him for a week, only to drop out after two days.

But other people work eighteen hours a day. The real issue is what we do in those hours.

What Henry does is drive himself hard to pass along the message he constantly repeats, like a mantra, behind podiums—sometimes a dozen times a day, including breakfasts, lunches, dinners, after-dinner talks and conference speeches—and lives every day in his work: "Deliver the scientific fact," he says in his insistent staccato. This is a man who delivers in person.

Henry Lee is a criminalist. Specifically, after retiring as Connecticut's Commissioner of Public Safety, he was appointed chief emeritus of the Connecticut Forensic Science Laboratory. He is a generalist in a world of specialists: While a blood-spatter expert may work with blood and blood alone for years, experimenting in it, testifying about it, even patenting machinery to examine it, Lee does blood beautifully—and a whole lot more. Criminalistics involves everything from initially recognizing something as evidence to collecting, preserving, identifying, individualizing and evaluating that evidence. It also includes reconstructing the events of the crime based on the evidence analysis and the interpretation of patterns at the crime scene.

And while nobody does it better, it might seem surprising that a criminalist is arguably the most recognizable man in the state of Connecticut—everywhere he goes he is stopped for a chat, an autograph, a picture, or to be given a plaque or a gift, or even to hoist a baby in his arms. But also around the world, in airports, hotels and restaurants, Henry is sought out by the public.

I have seen it happen time and again. Once, when he and I were flying together to examine bodies at a mass grave in Croatia, we changed planes in Frankfurt, only to be mobbed in the airport. Some people simply wanted to touch him.

Why? He solves mysteries—plain and simple—and that fascinates us. We marvel at it. We read millions of novels every year, watch hundreds of hours of television and movies, tear through the pages of magazine and newspaper articles about solving crime. This is the man who solves crime better than anyone else ever has. And he does so with grace and humility. American and European fans approach him wherever he goes, but that's nothing compared to what happens to him in Taiwan and China: There, they give him parades.

The first time around, the case of the disappearance of Helle Crafts ended in a mistrial. It was a tough case, after all—the first time anyone had been tried for murder in Connecticut without a body.

The case began right before Christmas 1986, when Richard

Crafts told neighbors that his wife, Helle, a flight attendant, had driven off after an argument. When she failed to show up for work, her coworkers reported their fears to the police. But without a body—the corpus delicti—no immediate charges could be filed. When Crafts finally filed a missing persons report after several weeks, that brought the case some public attention.

It was then that a snowplow driver remembered seeing a man fitting Crafts's description running a wood chipper near a body of water. The image stuck in the driver's memory because the chipping was being done at 3:30 A.M., during an unexpected snowstorm.

Speculation grew that Richard Crafts had killed his wife, cut up her body with a chain saw, placed the parts in plastic bags in a rented truck, driven to Lake Zoar and, using a rented wood chipper, chipped her body into mulch.

Henry immediately identified a body of water under a specific bridge that he wanted searched. He knew that currents had previously moved many things to that site. A chain saw was recovered from the water, from which he was able to lift a faint identification number that tracked the appliance back to Crafts, as had the rental of the wood chipper and the truck. That helped to complete the circumstantial evidence, but this was 1986: Advances in forensic sciences had brought us spectroscopic fiber analysis and "DNA fingerprinting," but jurors would need someone to tie together all that new science if they were to be expected to convict without a body.

It would take diligence and rigid scientific analysis to bring this case to conviction. For three weeks investigators searched the area where the chipper had been spotted, recovering and removing from the site what appeared to be wood chips and tissue.

Back at the lab, workers followed Henry's instructions and sorted the evidence into piles: leaves and other natural plant material in one, wood chips in another. Suspected tissue bits, bone fragments and hair went into other piles. It was tedious work, and it was only the beginning.

Thousands of analyses were made of the hairs and fibers alone: to separate human hairs from fibers, to divide human hairs according to the body parts from which they originated, to type the hair by race and categorize it as either pulled from skin or shed naturally, and then to examine the ends to determine whether the hairs were cut by scissors or by the blade of a wood chipper.

The wood chips were painstakingly examined, an attention to detail that resulted in the discovery of body fragments, including pieces of bone, a fingernail, a toenail, teeth and dental crowns, hair, clothing fibers and bits of the plastic bags. But even after this meticulous work, the total amount of body parts recovered by the police weighed only a few ounces.

All told, the prosecution's case, in what became known as the "Wood Chipper Murder," included expertise from across the spectrum of the sciences. For instance, Henry brought the body fragments to the New York State Police forensic science lab, where Dr. Lowell Levine was able to identify teeth fragments as belonging to Helle Crafts.

But teeth are not a body: Maybe she was alive with missing teeth or missing fingers. Asked to examine the bone fragments, I could identify one small fragment as coming from a skull bone. Bone fragments from the skull means the person is dead.

Henry went on to identify the human tissue on the chain saw as matching that in the mulch; strands of hair recovered at the scene as identical matches to those in a hairbrush in the Crafts' home; and fingernail polish from a shard of a human nail as a match to that found in a bottle in the Crafts' home.

Henry left nothing unexamined, including the wood itself.

He consulted the "wood man" of the University of Massachusetts, Amherst, R. Bruce Hoadley, who is well known in the forensic science world for being able to read the secrets of trees. Of course, he can identify trees the old-fashioned way—from leaves, bark, seeds and cones—but he can also analyze cellulose under the microscope to determine the type of tree the wood came from. These skills convinced Henry Lee to include Hoadley on the wood chipper case.

Hoadley was asked to identify the wood found on the ground at the site of the chipping, as well as the wood found in the back of the truck Crafts had rented to haul the chipper to his property. Under the microscope, the two sets of wood matched. He discovered that cut marks on some of the chips matched the blades of the chipper that Crafts had rented. This put Crafts at the crime scene and made the wood evidence.

Not since the Lindbergh murder case in the 1930s, in which a forestry expert identified which factory milled the wood used by the murderer to build the ladder he climbed to enter the home and kidnap the baby, has wood analysis proved so important in a case.

In all, nearly a hundred witnesses testified to their individual expertise. If there was any doubt about who is the finest criminalist in the world, it was dispelled when Henry pulled together the myriad scientific facts into testimony that reconstructed for the jury how Helle Crafts came to die and what became of her body.

It took almost three years of painstaking work, but in 1989, Richard Crafts was convicted of the murder of his wife. He is serving a fifty-year sentence.

The birth of the modern crime lab can be traced directly to fiction. Sir Arthur Conan Doyle was a physician and keen observer of his patients' abnormalities. He was a splendid writer, as well, and when he created Sherlock Holmes, he also imprinted on popular culture the idea that when the elements of science are coupled with applied logic, crimes can be solved. Doyle also knew that the way to brand the concept in the public's hearts and minds was to package the science in the form of a uniquely fascinating man.

After all, it had worked before, in Charles Dickens's *Bleak House,* published in 1853. In that novel, Inspector Bucket personified all that amazed the public about Scotland Yard.

By the time Doyle was writing, in the 1880s, London had had a police force for fifty years and the detectives of Scotland Yard since 1842. Starting in the 1860s, those detectives had added crime scene analysis to their toolbox of skills, and the forensic sciences took a great leap forward. But when Doyle captured it all in the form of Holmes, he did more than just sell books. One avid fan was Edmund Locard, who was reportedly greatly influenced by the writing and went on to build the world's first forensic laboratory in France in 1910.

The idea of crime labs spread throughout the world. In 1932, the Federal Bureau of Investigation opened its first lab under its first director, J. Edgar Hoover.

Six years later Chang-Yuh Lee was the thirteenth—and last—child born to a wealthy family in Ru-Ko, a small village in mainland China's Jiangsu province. When he was six, his mother, An-fu Wang-Lee, fled wartime China and went to Taiwan with her children. Her husband, Ho-Ming Lee, was to meet his family there the following year. He made it only as far as the Shanghai harbor, where his ship was shelled. He died in the attack, and the family fell into poverty.

"Many nights, I went to bed without food," recalls Lee. It is timely that the talk has turned to food, since he is on his way to a lunchtime lecture. Later he will make two dinner speeches at opposite ends of Connecticut. His record is seventeen talks in one day; he carries several of his twenty different slide shows in his car trunk at all times.

His lunchtime talk takes place at the Aqua Turf Club, at the twenty-fifth annual conference of the Connecticut River Valley's chapter of the American Industrial Hygiene Association. The group's representative appears visibly relieved to see Henry swoop into the allotted parking space at the catering hall, but less than happy when the criminalist emerges and walks toward him carrying a box.

"Slides?" the man asks nervously.

"Yes."

The simple response triggers a flurry of activity. Minutes later the man is back. There is no projector. Two words into the apology Dr. Lee whips out his cell phone, and within fifteen minutes, a projector arrives by trooper transport. The traveling show can go on.

"Never cave in," Henry says, explaining everything from getting a slide projector delivered to a catering hall in the suburbs to extracting a DNA sample from a sitting president. "Don't let emotion or media pressure or public sentiment or personal vendetta or personal feeling dictate a case," he says. "If you cave in, you have a problem."

Not caving was a sturdy ethic in the impoverished Lee household during the family's time in Taiwan. Despite their circumstances, eleven of his siblings went on to receive graduate degrees. For his part, Henry applied to the Taiwan Police College, considered then and now to be one of the finest schools for police training in the world. For a family in such poverty, it certainly helped that the tuition was free. He graduated at the top of his class and was rewarded within three months by becoming the youngest police captain in the history of the Taiwan force.

But there was a problem. His hours were driving his officers crazy. He did nothing but work. He had no girlfriend to encourage him to take leisure time. So one day when a smart, beautiful national basketball and track star named Margaret Song came into the department with an overextended visa from Sarawak (now part of Malaysia) hoping to rectify her visitor status, his officers insisted that she must deal directly with their captain. She did. She and Captain Lee were married in 1962. Eventually, though, Margaret wanted to return home, and Henry quit the police department and became a reporter for a Chinese-language newspaper in Malaysia.

He knew only four words of English in 1965 when he traveled to America with fifty dollars in his pocket, Margaret by his side and his dreams to complete a Ph.D. in science in his heart. After arriving in New York, he worked as a waiter in a Chinese restaurant, a groundskeeper, a stock boy, a medical laboratory technician and a martial arts instructor, and he earned a forensic science degree from John Jay College of Criminal Justice. The couple had two children. By 1975 Henry had earned his Ph.D. in biochemistry from New York University, and the family moved to Connecticut. Henry accepted a faculty position at the University of New Haven, becoming, in effect, a one-man forensic science department.

He soon started volunteering his services to the Connecticut State Police. At the time, their crime laboratory amounted to little more than a polygraph machine, a fingerprint kit and a microscope, all housed in a four-drawer file cabinet in a stripped-down men's room. In those days, it was pretty much the state of the art for the police lab.

In the twenty-five years since, Henry has taken on positions with five offices, culminating in his present position as chief emeritus of the Connecticut Forensic Science Laboratory. Along the way he has read and studied everything he can in the sciences. "Never waste time," he says. As a result, he knows all he can about everything from blood, bugs and ballistics to toxicology, accident reconstruction and jurisprudence, to name only a few areas of expertise. He also knows how to lobby for funds, develop an academic department, give a talk to any group at any time on any topic in any of the forensic sciences—including a whopper of a motivational talk to high school students (he books this one six years in advance)—in any of the six languages he speaks, as well as how to stay focused under enormous pressure.

Under his guidance the Connecticut State Police Crime Lab has grown to more than 38,000 square feet, employing more than forty people and housing many millions of dollars' worth of the latest equipment. Each year it conducts nearly half a million examinations and tests on physical evidence and is visited by people from all over the world who come to see the model crime lab—the best in the world, the house that Henry Lee built.

We met right after Henry moved to Connecticut. I quickly learned why Henry is so effective at a crime scene and how his attention to detail sets him apart. We were investigating a shooting death to determine whether it was homicide, suicide or accident. He was carefully examining the blood spatter and brain tissue on the bedding and floor through his huge magnifying glass.

After a while I asked, "What are you looking for?"

"I don't know," he replied. "But I'll tell you when I find it."

In a life of few advantages, Henry has one that has served him well: In his ability to synthesize being cop, newspaper reporter, teacher, scientist and multinational figure, he has lost none of the qualities of each and brings all of them to his work. In the course of his career—and in many ways because of it—the lab has morphed from police lab to crime lab to what we call it today, forensics laboratory. And as a result, much like the connection between the fictional Sherlock Holmes and the birth of the crime lab, there is an indisputable link between the astonishing Henry Lee and forensic sciences practiced all over the world today. Except this time, the man is for real.

Five years ago a woman in a small town in Alaska began her day by stepping into her white cotton underpants. Now those same panties are under the magnifying glass held by Dr. Henry Lee, having come the distance in the U.S. mail.

"Seams are intact, wrinkles in elastic typical with washing in hot water, slight separations, label all worn, no damage," Lee says to his assistant in the lab. Inch by inch, they will review the panties, cutting tiny samples from several spots that long ago were circled and numbered and presumably tested for semen and blood.

Then the panties will go back into one of many evidence bags shipped in a large, tattered supermarket box that looks nothing like what you would expect to see in a high-tech lab such as this. It would be easy to think that a box like this shouldn't be here— should be ashamed to be here—touched up as it is at the seams and corners with odd and jagged pieces of tape, stuffed with mismatched crumpled brown bags. But Henry says, as he might in court, "Everything equal."

And if the man is the medium and the science is the message, then that little motto is his brand: Everything equal. It is a card he has played from the start, institutionalizing it in Connecticut, in fact, when much to the consternation of many in law enforcement, he opened the lab to both prosecutors and defense attorneys, allowing both sides to inspect the evidence and confer with him.

It is this sense of equality that makes him so good: Nothing— not a rock star, a rich man, a president, not power or threats, undue influence, obvious sets of circumstances, pleading or begging— alters his consistent, simple rule of looking at everyone and everything the same. That and the fact that he says what he thinks.

Perhaps it was Henry's experience as a newspaper reporter that taught him what makes a good quote. He once told defense attorney Jack Litman, who had retained his services to consult on the case of the "Preppy Murderer," Robert Chambers, that his client was "guilty as hell." Litman didn't ask him to testify. When a prosecutor in the William Kennedy Smith rape trial asked Lee, as a defense witness, why he used a silk handkerchief to see whether the lawn at the Palm Beach Kennedy estate had left grass stains on the alleged victim's clothing, he replied in his Mandarin English, "Usually I do not carry panties. I carry handkerchief." And then there is the memorable line Henry uttered under oath at the O.J. Simpson trial when looking at some contaminated blood evidence: "Something wrong."

In his lunchtime slide talk to the industrial hygienists he is no less quotable. Describing a photograph of a footwear impression on the door of a murder victim: "Front door kicked in. Very high kick. Either teenagers or Bruce Lee. Use logic." Observing a photo of a crime scene investigation showing Henry squatting and the officers standing around: "Just like highway construction: one person work, all others observe." At another crime scene investigation: "Crime scene just like family reunion. Without coffee and donuts, we cannot do our job." Accompanying a shot of Monica Lewinsky's stained Gap dress: "Three hundred reporters shouting at me that morning, 'Dr. Lee, Dr. Lee, you have dress?' I tell them I never owned dress in my life." Again, on the Gap dress: "In Clinton's dictionary DNA stands for 'Do Not Ask.'" When swamped by reporters at a Washington airport en route to investigate the Vincent Foster suicide: "I say, 'Dr. Lee? No, I Mr. Wong. All Chinese look alike.'" And when not wanting to be quoted, he'll simply say, "Don't speak English."

He launches into the heart of his noontime speech. "In 1970, motive, means, opportunity were how we solve murders and between ninety to ninety-five percent victims know assailant. In 1980, drive-by. Serial murder. Reason profile only work in mystery movies. Profile of a rapist. What does he look like?"

Henry scans the group for one of his hosts.

"Stand up, Mark. Say hello to everybody."

There is general laughter as Henry continues.

"Statistic ninety-nine point nine percent male. One-tenth percent female. So Marty," he says, calling out to another host, "you want her phone number, right?"

More laughter.

He even knows to build rewards into the talk. Before he left his packed but orderly Meriden, Connecticut, office, he stuffed his pockets with handfuls of something from a drawer. Now, an hour later, he has one hand in a pocket as he continues his talk.

"What's the average age of a rapist?" he asks the group.

People shout out ages; one says, "Eighteen to twenty-eight."

"You close. Come up here," says Henry as he clarifies the point. "Average age rapist, sixteen to thirty-two," he says, looking the middle-aged man up and down, "but with Viagra you can still do it." He reaches into his pocket and hands him a Junior Trooper badge. He will give away eight during this session, seamlessly moving toward his crescendo with a message and a reward, a message and a reward, and then the big message.

"Early 1990s, we united the community using witnesses. And the community rallied behind us. Today, no one come forward to testify. Why? The system failed them: Become a witness, get punished. We lose public trust. With forensic work you cannot afford to make mistakes because all you have is the public trust, and if you violate it, you lose it. One-chance marriage. Some have two chances, three, with marriage. With forensic science crime scene— one chance—you mess up, it's gone."

While the humor and the badges may seem only to have served the purpose of mitigating the shock of viewing bloody crime scenes and dead bodies right before lunch, in fact, they also help make the subject enjoyable. A spoonful of humor and the overall message seem to go down well with the group. They applaud wildly and then whisk Henry into lunch when the talk is done.

Each day begins in the same way and in the same place it ended: in the morning and in the lab. After working in his lab, he'll go to bed at 1 A.M., and then he will get up a few hours later and go right back. There are three labs in Henry's life: the one he keeps at his home on the Connecticut coast, the state police crime lab in Meriden and the Henry C. Lee Institute of Forensic Science at the University of New Haven.

At 5 A.M. he is in his home lab, logging some of the 120 working hours he puts in each week. Here, he will look at private-practice evidence, although since he is almost always awake, the police come by at all hours with whatever needs his immediate attention.

By 7 A.M. he is in his car, heading north. By 7:30 he is in Meriden. At some point in the day he will be on the University of New Haven campus, today only to drop off a check, another of the countless donations he makes from his defense work. As if in his own defense, he says, "How many meals can a man eat in one day? Three. How many houses can he sleep in? One. I give the money away." And he does, to one of the forensic labs or sometimes directly to a struggling student. No one is quite sure just how much he has given over the years, but it is most of what he has earned in the hundreds of cases outside of Connecticut on which he has consulted—and, yes, since everybody always asks, this includes the fees he received in the O.J. Simpson case.

After his third high-speed trip to Meriden today, he will return a stack of phone calls, answer e-mails and review plans with a young firefighter and aspiring portraitist who wants to capture Henry on canvas. (A blur? A smear? A puff of smoke, perhaps? The fireman-painter laughs off the suggestions and then looks puzzled, but he doesn't know Henry yet.) Then he will open the file books on some of Lee's three hundred active and eight hundred cold cases.

In one, gruesome crime scene photos appear one after the other, page after page, revealing the death of a woman whose husband maintains that she killed herself with a rifle. Her relatives disagree. Among the crime scene notes are the written observations of the responding officer, including yet another quotable line, complete with attribution, from the scene.

"Keep Mind Open," it reads. "Dr. Lee."

Six
SCENES

Being a juvenile delinquent has served me well all my life. At six years of age, after that determination was made, I was sent away from my home in the Bronx to live at the Hawthorne Reform School in Westchester county, New York, run by the Jewish Board of Guardians. It was teeming with kids in trouble, most of whom were products of unhappy marriages.

After life in the Bronx in the 1930s, moving to a Jewish reform school in Westchester was like going to the country on vacation, despite the fact that I was in the youngest bunk, sharing the house with thirty other like-minded peers.

We called our houseparents Mom and Pop Ogara. Mom Ogara taught me many things, among them the vast array of rules that comprise proper table manners, but perhaps more important, she shared with me a fascination with Bellevue Psychiatric Hospital. She came by knowledge of both naturally, as a result of her work, and she took equal delight in talking about them.

In her telling, Bellevue was one of the wonders of the world, where great people practiced excellent medicine and cured the less fortunate of ills that society had only begun to understand. Early on, I set my sights on seeing this wonder after being "reformed" and returned home. I traveled there alone by train when I was thirteen. I simply stood outside of Bellevue Psychiatric and marveled at this huge, dark, fortresslike structure with its windows guarded by dark metal bars. Carried by the East River flowing behind it, the voices of the patients calling out the windows skittered across the water. I stood there, taking it all in, and vowed to go inside someday.

The awe remained, and years later I began medical school at New York University, whose pathology building was next door to Bellevue Psychiatric. It was only a matter of months before I made it from anatomy class down to the Bellevue morgue, shared by the city's medical examiner, where I began helping out as a medical student and then moonlighting during my internship and residency. I couldn't understand why everyone didn't want to work there. I loved that morgue.

My first paid official job was as an assistant medical examiner, which essentially entailed going to scenes of death. The job paid twenty-five dollars for an eight-hour shift and required fitting the work in between my hours as a resident. Many nights this meant sleeping at the morgue, which I did happily, in a little room next to the old-fashioned hospital switchboard. When the phone rang, I took down the information and went off to the scene.

During the first years I was sent to scenes of natural death only. A regular medical examiner covered the homicides, which at the time totaled fewer than 500 per year in New York City. By 1970, it was 2,000. Now it is down to under 700.

As a medical resident I found myself treating sick people during the day—drug addicts, battered children, suicide attempts, all on hospital turf, in hospital gowns, all very sanitized—while during the evening I would be on medical examiner call, up most of the night, going to a Bowery flophouse to examine a dead alcoholic in his filthy three-dollars-per-night cubicle, his uninterested peers sleeping nearby. I came to realize that, in some places, death was just another event of the night and day.

Then one night while I was still an intern, the two worlds met. Someone I had seen as a patient turned up dead. That day I had assisted the surgical resident in closing the cut wrists of a woman who had come into the psychiatric service, having made a bloody attempt at killing herself. It seemed more of a cry for help than a real attempt. I watched, fascinated, as the resident doctor carefully swabbed the cuts on her wrists and stitched them up: He treated the wounds as if it were the razor's fault. That same evening, working at the medical examiner's office, I attended the same woman, after she had been discharged from the hospital and jumped to her death off the roof of her building.

During that experience, it became apparent to me that all too often, as physicians, we focus on the physical problem rather than on what causes that problem: The problem was not the cut wrist; the problem was that she had been terribly depressed. After viewing the body, I walked around the dead woman's apartment and saw the circumstances of her life—the empty fridge, the note she left recounting how her husband had left, that she didn't know how to care for her two children, about previous suicide attempts—and for the first time, the scene and the death and the backstory fit in a way that only someone who works the whole story can see in its totality.

Looking at the needle tracks on someone's arms gives a forensic pathologist insight into a family situation that was in trouble for long periods of time—the lying, the inadequate health care, problems on the job. But going to the scene shows the investigator the shooting gallery in the protected doorway leading to the roof, the dead man huddled in its frame, surrounded by empty heroin bags and old needles left by him and his cronies, who scattered after the death. It tells us a story about how these people lived, as well as the desperateness of their situation.

There is no substitute for visiting and working the scene.

As interns and medical students we learned to ask the patient for the history: Where does it hurt? Did it ever hurt like that before? Do you smoke? Drink? Any past surgeries? But when we see a dead body, we can't ask such questions, which is why we have to learn to read the body at the scene, if possible, and on the autopsy table.

On the table, we read what we see. At the scene, we poke around, looking at the empty whiskey bottles, what is on the stove or in the fridge, whether there is digitalis or insulin in the medicine chest, sleeping pills or Prozac, cocaine or heroin. And all of that helps us decide whether the death is natural or unnatural and whether an autopsy is warranted. We can't do autopsies out of interest only. There must be a compelling factor that makes society's needs outweigh the family's right not to have one performed.

Getting information from a crime scene has its own history. Several times that history has taken great lurches forward.

Late in the nineteenth century, the unsolved cases of Jack the Ripper were horribly embarrassing to the home office in London. The usual methods employed to catch criminals were not working. The result was the establishing of police detectives and a forensic pathologist dedicated to work in criminal investigation. The fact that the Ripper was never caught served as a major factor in pressing for the recognition of the importance of forensic science.

One hundred years later, it would be a double homicide in Brentwood, California, that would once again fix the world's attention on the importance of forensic science. And just as Jack the Ripper had called attention to the need to specialize in homicide investigation, the O.J. Simpson murder case would focus the world's attention on the importance of protecting the crime scene.

My connection to the O.J. Simpson case began in 1974, when

William Kunstler cross-examined me in a trial in the Bronx. He was defending a person who had been accused of holding up someone in the subway. The prosecutor's theory was that during the armed holdup, an off-duty cop happened onto the scene and pulled out a gun, prompting the accused to run up a set of stairs while shooting at the off-duty officer. Then a tragic coincidence occurred: A uniformed cop showed up, the accused yelled that some wacko was shooting at him and the uniformed cop shot and killed the off-duty police officer.

Kunstler did his best defending the accused, cross-examining me on the stand and bringing out the evidence to support his client; and although the man was initially found guilty, he was later set free after appeal.

Then in 1990, Marlon Brando's son was arrested for shooting a man in his father's Los Angeles home. Christian Brando, who was thirty-two at the time of the shooting, told police that he had accidentally killed Dag Drollet, the boyfriend of his twenty-year-old half sister, Cheyenne, after the pregnant Cheyenne had complained to him that evening of being slapped around by her 6 foot 3 inch, 270-pound lover.

Christian maintained that he had confronted Drollet with a .45-caliber handgun, which went off when Drollet tried to wrestle it away from him. There were reportedly no witnesses: Marlon Brando, sixty-six, his forty-eight-year-old wife, Tarita Teriipia, and Cheyenne had been in other parts of the hillside house when the shots rang out. The story was that Marlon had rushed to the den and attempted mouth-to-mouth resuscitation before and after phoning 911 for assistance.

The cops arrested Christian on the spot. Two days later he was arraigned on first-degree murder and lesser charges, to which he pleaded not guilty. The elder Brando had called Kunstler minutes after the shooting. They had previously worked together for Native Americans, beginning with the 1974 defense of Indian leaders Russell Means and Dennis Banks for illegally occupying

Wounded Knee in South Dakota. Kunstler showed up to plead for Christian's release on bail, citing letters from supporters, including Jack Nicholson. But Deputy DA Steven Barshop argued that the killing was premeditated, claiming the angle of the wound proved that Drollet had been shot from above while lying down on the couch, not while in a struggle. Bail was denied.

The boyfriend had been killed by an in-and-out wound of the chin and neck. But no bullet had been recovered, either in the dead man or at the scene. Brando wanted to bring in a forensic pathologist to have a second look. Kunstler had suggested me because he thought my testimony had been very fair in our previous dealings, so I flew to Los Angeles to do a second autopsy on Drollet. The thought was that maybe the bullet was still in the body. It wasn't.

So I asked to go back to the scene, Brando's house on Mulholland Drive. That is where I met Bob Shapiro, later an O.J. Simpson defense lawyer, who had been retained by the Brando family as local counsel. We went in, and I met Marlon Brando, his wife and a bunch of the kids.

I advised Brando that we were going to have to look at the scene, which, it turned out, had not been secured by the police. People had been coming and going in and out of that room since the police had left. The bloodstained furniture had been moved to a shed on the property, which meant we had to take it all out to inspect it, the thought being that perhaps the bullet was embedded in the couch. It wasn't.

When I went into the room where the shooting occurred, the first thing I saw was a thick shag rug. I shook my head, knowing what the problem was. Experience has taught me that there are two places cops hate to look for bullets: in feces and in shag rugs. Here we had the latter. You don't see a neat bullet hole in a shag rug.

Where the bullet landed was very important in this case. The police had already given out their version of the story on day one. When they arrived, the first 911 responder had said he found

Drollet lying on his back on the couch, with the television on, and the channels flipping continuously, as though the man was scanning for a favorite program. In one hand, he held a cigarette lighter. But he was dead, having been shot once in the chin. The police assumed and announced that he had been shot while in the same position in which he had been found, which was an unwarranted assumption. Everybody falls down after they are shot: Gravity affects all of us the same.

So, I got down on my hands and knees and felt around in the rug as the senior Brando walked on it, feeling through the shag with his bare feet. And there it was, under the rug, nice and flat, just the way it should be. When a bullet goes through a carpet, hits a marble floor like the one that was there and then skids along under the rug, it produces a very specific type of ricochet I've seen before and since.

Brando and I looked at this bullet together, its one surface very shiny, where it had struck the marble floor under the rug. Shapiro called the police, and when they arrived I spoke to the sergeant. "Hey," I said, "this is a very high-profile case. How could they give up the crime scene without finding the bullet?"

He looked at me and said, sadly, "Doc, if you got people doing lousy jobs, they can't suddenly do a good job just because it's a high-profile case."

He was absolutely right. At the time, I had no idea how prophetic that line would prove to be.

Since the 1960s, forensic science crime investigation has evolved beyond its dependence on interrogation and confession. At that time, 85 percent of murders involved family members, loved ones or friends. In the 1970s, stranger murders increased, and we became fascinated with motive and opportunity. By the 1980s, killing didn't make the sense it once did because in only 60 percent of the homicides was there a relationship between the killer and the victim. Suspect profiling emerged as an investigative tool. The problem with profilers is that they always pontificate on the obvious, and they usually lack on-the-scene experience. They develop profiles that a good detective often has learned on the street: Rapist-murderers are almost always males, between eighteen and thirty-five years old, who live within a twenty-five-mile radius of their victims. That's good to know, but it still doesn't tell you who did it.

Trace evidence burst on the scene in the late 1980s with the development of DNA. The term *DNA fingerprinting* was coined by British geneticist Alec Jeffreys. Now the technology is used to convict suspects as well as to exonerate those wrongly accused.

DNA, which stands for deoxyribonucleic acid, is present in the nucleus of all of our cells. It resembles a long, spiraling ladder. Combinations of carbon, hydrogen, oxygen, nitrogen and phosphorous atoms form the sugar-phosphate sides of the ladder. The rungs are made up of pairs of four nucleic acids—adenine, thymine, guanine and cytosine. Our genes are basically the biochemical directions spelled out by the specific sequence of pairs of these acids.

Ninety-nine percent of our genes are identical among humans. It is the other one percent that makes us unique. Although everyone shares the same sets of genes that determine physical characteristics and manufacture necessary proteins and enzymes, large sections of our DNA contain repeating sequences of nucleic acids that have no known purpose. But this DNA does serve a very important function when applied to identification: It varies from person to person. Within these regions of unknown purpose lie repeating sequences of nucleic acids called microsatellites. Specifically, the numbers of repeats, or polymorphisms, vary from one individual to another. The patterns of repeats make up the DNA fingerprint.

DNA testing is performed by chopping up several repeating areas with special enzyme probes that snip DNA at the same corresponding spaces. The fragmented DNA is sorted according to the size of the pieces and then counted, since at any given site one person may have twelve repeats while another may have fifteen. Several sites are compared. Matching patterns presumably come from the same person. To achieve the greatest accuracy, and therefore to make it onto the stand in the courts, the expert must calculate the chances that any two people could coincidentally share the same patterns.

Material that may contain DNA is collected at the crime scene: Blood, semen, saliva and hair torn from the scalp are the main substances we look for that can help crime solving immeasurably. We read about spectacular cases—DNA testing that proved the paternity of Thomas Jefferson's offspring by his slave Sally Hemings, or that freed innocent men on death row. What does not make the headlines is usually some of the best science. When DNA testing is done quickly, it can result in a quick confession. We may not hear about these cases, because they never go to trial. Also, this kind of testing can link seemingly unrelated crimes to the same perpetrator and generate leads at the beginning of an investigation. It is a national disgrace that because of lack of funds in many places—New York City being one of them—rape kits are not routinely tested immediately, but instead are kept until a suspect is found and are then tested. In other words, scientific analysis is done backward.

Around the country, detectives are being instructed to pick up chewing gum, tissues, bandages, cigarette butts, soda cans and other items previously considered throwaways at crime scenes. Drinking cups offered to potential suspects during questioning are spirited away for DNA comparison to anything found at the scene. DNA can be obtained from blood, semen, hair, saliva, mucus and skin cells.

And so, in the 1990s, what we learned from DNA is the value of protecting and collecting trace evidence at the scene. No trace, no DNA. Simple as that. Trace brings other things on its own, of course, but DNA is, by far, the most distinguishing difference from person to person. Because of that reliability, juries are often more influenced by DNA results than by more traditional evidence such as fingerprints, handwriting or even eyewitnesses.

At the turn of the century we see the increased use of artificial intelligence. We have live-scan fingerprinting techniques, portable digital microscopes, lasers, every alternative light system imaginable to expose every human excretion, DNA typing, microchip DNA, instrumentation and automation, the capacity to beam by satellite the image from a crime scene right back to an expert to advise investigators what to look for and, of course, e-mail and voice mail. All of it is available to law enforcement to utilize in recognizing and reconstructing the information needed to put the case together. We can study blood-pattern evidence, blood spatter, bullet trajectory, powder residue, casing ejection, fire burn, glass fracture; we can study clothing, and interview, analyze and autopsy all we want.

But there is one thing we cannot change, and that is human nature. Investigators often say that the ideal piece of evidence is the murderer's print in the victim's blood. But if no one collects it, that evidence is lost. All this burgeoning science is only as good as the hands that use it.

The murders of Nicole Brown Simpson and Ronald Goldman occurred on June 12, 1994. The first call to me came from Bob Shapiro on Thursday, June 16, close to midnight. He asked me for the best criminalist I knew. To me, the obvious answer was Henry Lee.

The next day—five days after the murders—Henry Lee and I arrived at the home of Robert Kardashian in an affluent part of Los Angeles. O.J. Simpson was in seclusion there, scheduled to give himself up to the LAPD that day at noon. We were to examine him before they did. Saul Faerstein, a forensic psychiatrist was also present, as was Bob Shapiro. The police did not know where Simpson was.

Henry and I asked Simpson to strip to his shorts. When he did, I had two clear impressions: first, that he was much thinner than I expected, and second, that he had a healing cut on one hand, but no other marks of a struggle on him. And after only moments together, I reached a conclusion: He was very depressed. The body posture and the lack of affect that are hallmarks of suicidal risk were quite obvious.

We photographed Simpson and took hair samples, then conferred with the psychiatrist. Henry and I advised the psychiatrist that we were convinced Simpson should be kept under suicidal precautions. His belt and shoelaces, as well as anything else he could use to hurt himself, should be taken from him. We had not quite finished our examination in the time allotted when several calls back and forth to the police occurred. They demanded to know our whereabouts so they could pick up their suspect. They were tired of waiting, it seemed, and did not want to be told that the deadline would not be met. They also declared that they had an arrest warrant. In the earlier telephone calls, Shapiro had not disclosed O.J.'s whereabouts. However, when the police said they had an arrest warrant, Shapiro immediately told the police where we were.

Henry and I then walked from the room toward a large picture window overlooking the driveway, where we could watch for the arrival of the police. We were told that O.J. was saying good-bye to his girlfriend in the bedroom nearby.

Any number of things may have happened after that, but what I know for certain is that we had examined and photographed Simpson, that we had been interrupted, that the police had shown up, that O.J. Simpson was nowhere to be found and that all of a sudden, Henry and I went from being the experts flown in from the East Coast to being potential accessories to the escape. Thankfully for us, one of the cops recognized Henry from a lecture he had recently given the police department, and everyone appropriately began to focus their attention on the escapee.

The Los Angeles Police Department's failure to protect the crime scene happened in much the same way: People rushed in, made assumptions and made mistakes. I didn't see any evidence planted at the crime scene. No one had to. The police and other visitors tragically and inadvertently brought in and took away trace evidence on their feet, on their clothing and with their own hands.

The first hour of a crime scene is critical. In fact, the first person at a crime scene can change the entire direction of an investigation. Think for a minute of the JonBenet Ramsey case: A call was made reporting a kidnapping, and the local police, believing what they had been told by the caller, and being inexperienced in homicide detection, rushed in and literally walked all over what at one time was a scene filled with valuable clues.

The first person arriving at the crime scene is usually a passerby or a relative who does all manner of things to the body in an effort to revive it. A person discovering a body might flip it over, slap the face, pump the chest, take the pulse, even perform mouth-to-mouth resuscitation—all in a struggle to preserve life. But in doing that, the person changes the location and condition of the body, which the arriving police may not fully appreciate.

All too often, however, when the police arrive, the lowest-ranking and least-experienced officer is assigned to set up the perimeter protecting the crime scene. An experienced crime scene investigator knows that the first hour of a scene is critical and that in those sixty minutes the evidence can either be protected or destroyed. It all depends on the perimeter established.

It is the job of the first police officer on the scene to set up a perimeter through which only the necessary homicide detectives, laboratory personnel and medical examiners should be allowed to pass. Over the years I have seen crime scenes contaminated by mayors and their out-to-dinner guests, DAs who keep police scanners near their beds so they can show up at as many crime scenes as possible and all kinds of unneeded people who try to come and hover over homicide scenes. It shouldn't be allowed.

One way to keep mayors and other VIPs on the other side of the yellow tape is to set up two perimeters: one surrounding the scene of the crime, which can be entered by only several key people solely for the purpose of evidence collection, and another, farther back from the actual scene, for the VIPs.

Outside that second perimeter should be the press and the general public—inevitable observers, especially in high-profile cases. Everyone who enters either perimeter should be listed in a police logbook, thus making them part of the permanent record.

As trace evidence becomes more and more identifiable, analyzable and important, protective gear should be worn at all crime scenes. This includes gloves, hair nets, booties and protective coveralls.

By their own account, no protective gear was used by any of the initially responding police officers entering the scene of the Simpson-Goldman murders. During the Simpson trial, when prosecutor Marcia Clark was questioning Detective Philip Vannatter, he testified that as an old-time detective, his generation did not wear hair nets and booties. It just isn't done, he said.

This thinking has to change. A single hair out of place can destroy the value of a crime scene and will be challenged by the opposing counsel. Hair nets, booties and gloves do not seem too much to ask when justice is at stake.

The lack of protective covering at the Simpson-Goldman homicide scene also resulted in bloody shoe prints all over the area, most of which, after long investigation, turned out to have been made by the responding police officers. Even a quick review of the crime scene photos shows detectives, some in high heels, walking in the blood of the dead, sometimes walking from one body to the other—literally, from one crime scene into another.

This problem became a prosecution calamity when many of the detectives—Mark Fuhrman included—went from the bloody crime scene of the double homicide to the next suspected crime scene, the home of O.J. Simpson, walking about, again without booties, and thereby potentially transferring all sorts of trace evidence from the murder scene to the home of the accused.

There was also a piece of bloody paper on the ground near Nicole Simpson's head that never made it into evidence. Who knows what that piece of paper may have contained or where it went? Probably it left the crime scene on the sole of some unsuspecting detective's shoe. This transfer and contamination of trace evidence from one crime scene to another was surely inadvertent, but it quickly led to accusations of both tampering and planting of that evidence.

All the while the police were tramping through evidence at the scene of the double homicide, the bodies of Nicole Brown Simpson and Ronald Goldman lay out in the open, unexamined by a medical examiner. This was for the simple reason that nobody requested one.

This tragic mistake left unresolved the question of when the victims died. The measurements the medical examiner takes upon arriving at a scene can place the time of death accurately—the sooner after the death has occurred the better. In two hours, for instance, the jaw will stiffen. And the subtle differences leading up to the stiffening are best known to someone who has examined thousands of postmortem jaws.

Measuring the body for rigor mortis, degree of lividity and temperature has great value the sooner the body is seen, but little value once the body is removed to the morgue.

The medical examiner also must show up quickly at a crime scene to examine the body for trace evidence. Most police won't even touch a body. They are trained not to and most of them follow this training to the letter. And logically, this would mean that the medical examiner should be called immediately, since it is the responsibility of that office to identify, document, protect and collect evidence and to make sure none is lost en route to the morgue. Documentation is done by dictation, by writing and by photographs. Any ephemeral evidence is noted, collected and protected.

At the scene of the Simpson-Goldman murders, the medical examiner was treated as nothing more than a body-removal service. He was not even notified until ten hours after the bodies were found. By then, critical evidence had vanished forever.

The medical examiner would have gone into the residence and looked inside everything—medicine chests, garbage cans, cupboards, the refrigerator—and would have documented what was on the stove and in the sink, in search of anything of medical significance. All this would have been photographed and saved. This could have been something as seemingly insignificant as the dish of melting Ben & Jerry's ice cream found in Nicole Simpson's home. A lot was made of this at trial when it was revealed that while the cops saw it, no one photographed it. The medical examiner would have known to photograph it with the time noted and would have known to look for it in the stomach contents of the two victims to see if it might correlate with what was known about the last meal and when it was eaten. Even the melting time of the ice cream could have proven significant. And it is easily calculated by recreating the temperature and conditions of the night of the murders. That knowledge also would speak to the time of death, which, at trial, was never resolved.

The police are not accustomed to looking at pill bottles, food packages, alcohol bottles and the like and making the connection to the lives lived by the people who consumed their contents. Medical examiners are. It is what we do to document the scene properly and have a better, more informed chance of judging not only whether an autopsy should be done but what type and how extensive. Should all the foodstuffs in the entire gastrointestinal tract be preserved, for instance? Should the extremities be dissected? What about the face? Whether or not procedures beyond the normal basic autopsy should be done depends on what is at the crime scene and what might be relevant to answer questions that are bound to occur later on.

Ten hours later, however, much of this is moot.

The body of Nicole Brown Simpson was never viewed at the scene by a medical examiner. It was flipped over onto its back for removal to the morgue, where it was viewed, washed and photographed by a morgue photographer and then left for two days before an autopsy was performed. No proper trace evidence removal was ever performed. None could be: It had all been washed away.

Sloppy photographic work also plagued the Simpson case. Plenty of photographs were taken of the bodies at the scene, but none were taken inside the residence. Along with the dish of ice cream, these would have revealed any activity in or near the beds, any evidence of a struggle in the apartment or any number of things we cannot even imagine since we do not know what we are looking for until we find it. It's the basic rule of investigation: You never know what you are looking for.

The failures at the Simpson crime scene go on: failure to collect the blood drops on Nicole Brown Simpson's back; failure to examine and photograph the back gate (possibly the exit used by the killer), resulting in the accusation weeks later, when blood was found there, that it had been subsequently planted; failure to bag the hands of either victim; failure to perform a rape kit on either victim; and failure to protect the evidence, resulting in its loss or destruction, including that of one of the lenses in the eyeglasses Nicole Brown Simpson had left at the restaurant where Ronald Goldman worked and which he had been returning to her when they were both murdered.

Forensic science will prove to be of critical value only in a minority of cases. But we never know which ones. The majority of murders are still solved by old-fashioned police work: shoe leather and knocking on doors. Most cases will result in confessions or pleas long before trial. And most will not involve DNA comparison. But we don't know that going in. Who is to say what the next trial of the century will be? Or, equally important, the next trial of some poor, unknown defendant who deserves the same science that might exonerate him from a bad, biased or mistaken eyewitness?

We can't know. And one of the few positive results of the massive publicity of the Simpson case has been the focus on trace evidence and on the need to collect, preserve and test this evidence. The only way to do that is to protect every single crime scene against contamination.

Otherwise, we cannot say with all certainty that it was the perpetrator who either left something behind at the scene—a fingerprint, blood, semen, a shoe print, perhaps—or picked up something from the decedent and carried it away with him. In one of the cases I handled, the killer carried away his victim's fingernail in his trouser cuff. In another case, a single contact lens from a murdered girl was found in the backseat of the killer's car. Without worldwide publicity, dream teams, television, press corps, book deals, talk shows, or courtroom theatrics, both of those killers are in jail, based on the evidence that accused them of their crimes.

In this country, a defendant does not have to prove his or her innocence. Instead, our justice system requires that the prosecution prove guilt. The prosecutor has the burden to prove his or her case. The burden of proof, then, depends on how much you can rule in. In a murder case that means the defendant must be ruled in as the only possible killer. And it means that anything that is not done—failing to lift and identify blood samples from a dead woman's back, for instance—obstructs justice.

Seven

BUGS

The level, flat slab of the Midwest may be the place where the risky game of chicken was born. Here cars can race side by side or hurtle toward each other on a collision course at terrific speed without so much as the hint of an incline, a whisper of a curve or the shock of a stop sign. The road goes on forever until it meets another road at crisp right angles, only to go on again.

Houses are set back from the road and are sheltered by the only trees around: Large, leafy bowers hang the shade on the roofs that otherwise would bake in the Indiana sun. Go up in a plane and these little clots of houses and green trees appear as dots on the graph paper that is America's farmland. Box after box, rigid in their limits, limitless in their shades of yellow and green, the graph expands beneath you exponentially in all directions the higher you fly. Leaving the land behind becomes impossible: It simply grows under the wings of the plane until it is everywhere.

Indiana is the solid Midwest. There is no mistaking it. Here fireworks outlets brace the edges of the state, pork chops are on every restaurant menu, people drink Mr. Pibb and red pop and farmers drive the astonishing pieces of machinery that cultivate American agriculture. In the planting and harvesting seasons these machines roam the massive, soft fields that blanket the limestone base laid in the Upper Silurian Age.

Despite its name, Jasper County, Indiana, is bedrocked from end to end with that limestone. The county seat is a city called Rensselaer, a treed, cool oasis from the hot and dusty business of farming. In the middle of town is the Busy Bee ice cream stand by the Iroquois River. It opens in May, and its staff is good at giving directions to a well-known eight-hundred-acre farm just outside of town. You go east a ways; then, they will tell you, you start looking on the north side of the road. It turns out that the place is easy to find on an early summer night, distinguished, as it is, amid the threshers and the combines, by a slow moving, twenty-three-ton, steel-cleated World War II tank that is firing tennis balls into the dusk.

Dr. Neal Haskell, it seems, is spending a rare evening at home. As the only full-time professional forensic entomologist in the world, Dr. Haskell travels nearly all the time. But not this week. Every year at the beginning of the summer he runs a school. Law enforcement people from all over the world fly into Chicago or Indianapolis, then drive two hours to Rensselaer, to learn from the master about the ancient science of bugs on dead people.

Climbing out of the tank, he looks like nothing so much as a round peg in a small hole. Haskell, who is a professor of forensic science and biology at St. Joseph's College in Rensselaer, is a big boy, whose barrel-bellied shape stretches the slogans on his T-shirts into easy reading for the large-type set. This one reads MAGGOT POWER on the front and IT'S FUN TO PUT SNAP, CRACKLE AND POP INTO THE MOURNING on the back.

The beer he serves up out of the barn cooler, called "Old Scratch" lager, features a half-dog, half-flea mascot. The Dodge

Caravan SE parked next to the main house bears a license plate that reads MAGGOT. This man is dead serious—in a funny kind of way—about his bugs.

As a body starts to die something sends certain members of the bug world into a frenzy. Female blowflies have a keen sense of smell and from as far away as a mile and a half can smell the moments of death. Perhaps it is a gas discharged by bacteria in the gut. Perhaps it is something far more obscure.

The process was documented as early as 1235 A.D., when Sung Tz'u, a Chinese death investigator, wrote a book entitled *The Washing Away of Wrongs,* about the forensic sciences of the time. It contains what is probably the first written account of the use of bugs in determining criminal behavior. A slashing murder had occurred in a small Chinese village, and after the usual questioning of the locals, no suspect had been located. The local investigator then had all the villagers bring their sickles to an open spot and lay them out before the crowd. Flies landed on one of the sickles, probably because of the bits of the victim's tissue that remained on the instrument. The owner of the sickle broke down and confessed.

Experiments in 1668 by Francesco Redi essentially killed the widely held belief that rotting meat somehow spontaneously generated its own flies. The year 1855 saw the first use of insects as forensic indicators by a Westerner. When a baby's body was discovered behind the plaster mantle of a house in France, Dr. Bergeret d'Arbois performed an autopsy and determined that the assemblage of insects pointed to an earlier date, and thus previous occupants of the house, rather than those originally accused.

After that, it was a slow but inexorable series of steps to Rensselaer, Indiana, and Neal Haskell's summer bug school at the farm.

The night before things begin we are given our schedule. School will proceed pretty much like this: kill the pigs, watch for flies, look for maggots, do some experiments, drink some beers, have a pig roast.

At the heart of Rensselaer is the courthouse. It was erected in 1896, the year that Ohioan William McKinley beat out Nebras-kan William Jennings Bryan, the "boy orator," for president of the United States. The structure is Gothic in style, with strong Victo-rian flourishes. Inside are polished stone stairs and stenciled ceil-ings, all reflecting the organic colors of this part of the country. Stained glass staves of wheat give way on the upper floors to scales of justice set in the leaded windows.

Surrounding the courthouse square are the hallmarks of pros-perity of small town America. On the east side is the bank that lo-cals for years considered the Democratic bank (a Republican bank once shared the courthouse square but has been replaced). On the south side of the square is the fitness and tanning salon. Along the west flank is the Ritz cinema and an eatery called the City Office and Pub (the mayor's office used to be in the building). Heading north out of town on Route 231, you can pick up a copy of the Rensselaer *Republican,* the local newspaper, before arriving at the American Legion Hall. That's where bug school starts at 8 A.M. sharp.

Inside the hall, thirty-seven students, some still smelling of soap and showers, mill around, warming in the June morning. They are quiet and well groomed, the men all sporting the close-cropped hair of law enforcement, the seven women looking more like fringe-science, with assorted piercings and a smattering of tat-toos. The exception here is Laura, a Brooklyn-born FBI agent, whose dark hair is neat and trim and whose ankle is packing seri-ous heat. Her explanation of a recent use of "Cadavahdawgs . . . you know, *cadavahdawgs*" is met initially with a blank stare. It takes a classmate several attempts to comprehend. "Oh, cadaver dogs," he says, as the light of recognition ignites. In this part of the world her accent is rarer than a Waco fire maggot (which, inci-dentally, Dr. Haskell has in his celebrity maggot collection).

This is the bingo room of the American Legion Hall, as evi-denced by the ancient numbered light board and cage of num-

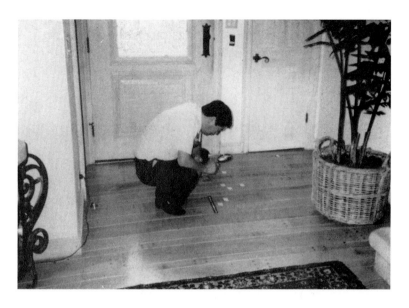

Dr. Henry Lee examining blood droplets that had been overlooked by police in the entranceway of O.J. Simpson's home.

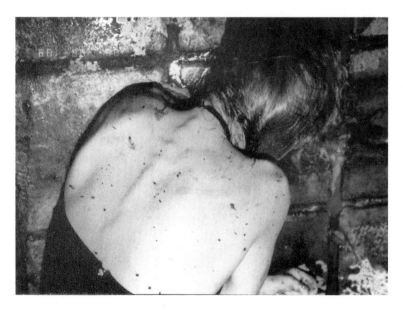

The low-velocity blood droplets on Nicole Simpson's back at the crime scene from a perpetrator that were not preserved and analyzed.

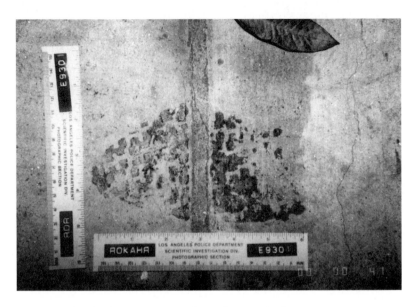

Perpetrator's bloody shoe print on the walkway at the Simpson crime scene.

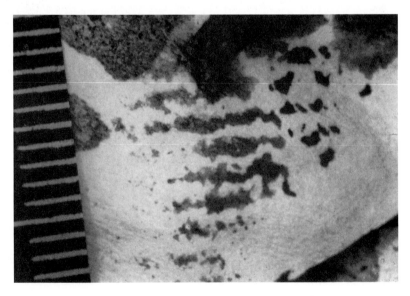

A different bloody shoe print of a perpetrator on the envelope containing the eyeglasses that Ron Goldman was returning to Nicole Simpson.

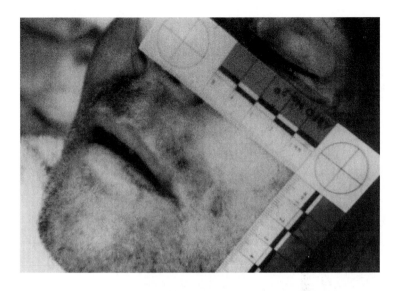

Ted Binion showing bruising and abrasions about the mouth, indicative of external pressure during suffocation.

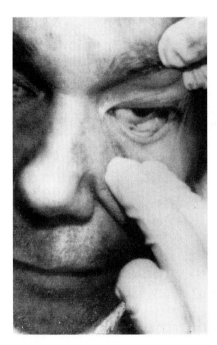

Petechial hemorrhage on Binion's inner eyelid from neck compression during suffocation.

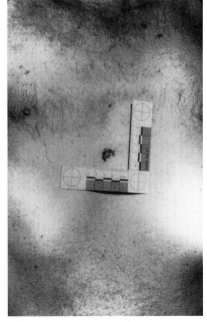

Shirt-button abrasions on Binion's chest from compression during burking-type suffocation.

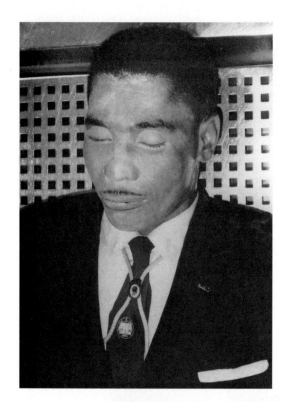

Medgar Evers, readily identifiable after removal from casket, twenty-eight years after burial.

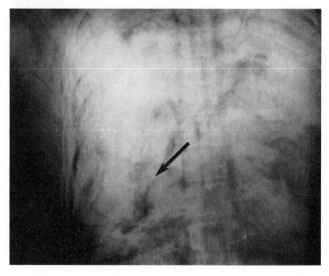

X ray of chest and abdomen showing small metal fragments (white) from .30-06 rifle bullet that struck Evers's rib while going through his body.

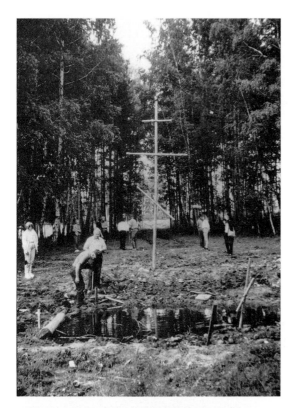

U.S. team examining secret burial site in Ural Mountains in Siberia from where Romanov remains, buried in 1918, were recovered.

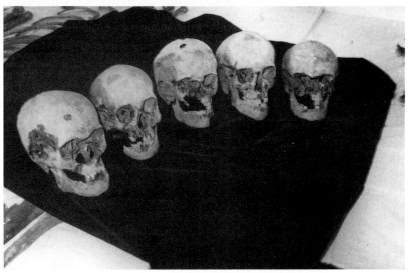

The recovered skulls of Nicholas, Alexandra, and the three older children, showing injuries from bullets, blunt rifle-butt impacts, and acid.

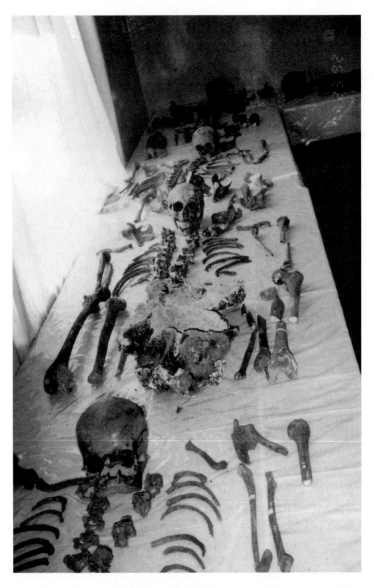

Skeletonized remains recovered from the burial site, at the Institute of Legal Medicine in Yekaterinburg, Russia.

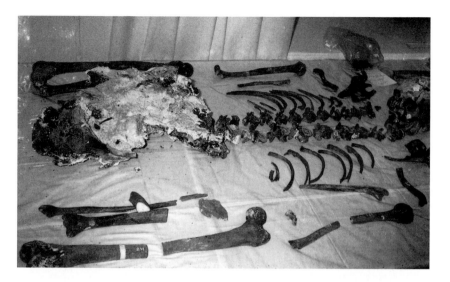

White adipocere formation—grave wax—still present on the remains of the murdered physician. (Long bones in the foreground had been cut for analysis of age.)

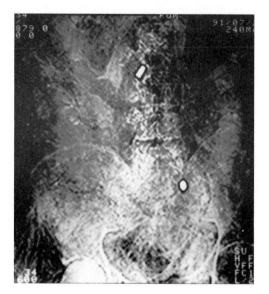

X ray of abdomen of Romanov physician showing two bullets, which, on removal, proved to be military ammunition from 1918.

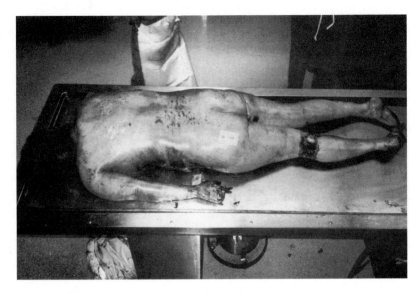

Body of a TWA Flight 800 passenger showing typically intact body despite freefall from 13,000 feet.

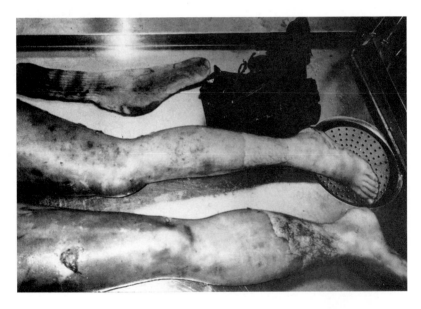

TWA 800 victim showing postmortem loss of the outer layer of skin from exposed areas of lower extremities due to jet-fuel burns.

bered balls to the left in front. On the upper right of the front wall of the hall are written the words of the preamble of the Constitution. Right under those words, Dr. Haskell sets up his maggot display. This consists of Schmidt boxes that store bugs, bottles with neoprene stoppers and a small but impressive insect collection. This is his traveling show. His lab, with thousands of bugs at varying stages of life and death, is in his mother's basement on one of the nicest streets in town.

Today Dr. Haskell is wearing a T-shirt whose sleeve reads NO FLIES ON ME. One of the students sets out to change that by offering the professor a great, shiny necklace of plastic beetles and flies in the electric colors of Mardi Gras beads. Strung amid the insects are tiny rubber maggots. Oh, Dr. Haskell loves this. This is a real treasure.

All too often people use the expression "larger than life" to describe people who really are not. Within the first few moments of bug school, it becomes apparent that Neal Haskell is, in fact, larger than life. He's enormous with it, delighted to be here, joyous in his enthusiasm about teaching and about maggots themselves.

"Good news, folks," he says, turning in the aisle between the rows of desks. "We've got maggots. We've got migrating maggots. We've got puparia." The twenty-five pigs that were killed last night have attracted the usual suspects. Most of the class seems to know this already: They were up early, checking on their pigs.

Laura was among the early risers. From her experiment she will write a paper discussing whether charring and burning flesh alters the time it takes for flies to alight on a corpse. Or, as she says, "When a perp tries to burn the bodies, we don't know how much delay that causes in the bugs." This paper will become a poster at the next American Academy of Forensic Sciences meeting in Reno, Nevada, in February. Knowing more about the question of bugs and charred flesh would have helped Dr. Haskell in a recent case in which someone tried to burn a body and left a perfect outline of it on the grass. That was helpful, and interesting, in terms of forensic botany. But the need for accuracy in forensic entomology demanded that Haskell know if the burning delayed the onset of the bugs and therefore delayed the well-known timetable of their activity. If so, that would help to determine the time of death.

That's one of the things certain bugs can do: They tell us when and where someone was killed, and they do it with exquisite accuracy that no man-made system will ever reproduce.

Dr. Haskell strolls around the room as he relates the details of a case he worked in Oklahoma, one of five hundred in his twenty-year career.

August in Stroud, Oklahoma, is a lot hotter than August in Rensselaer, Indiana, and flesh left out in the sun turns bad real fast. One morning a neighbor followed his nose across the street to the home of Aureliano Cisneros and his wife, Linda Howell. The stench emanating from a pile of junk in the driveway of their home had gone from being a curiosity to being a nuisance. And it was swarming with flies.

Underneath a pile of dresser drawers, blankets, suitcases and a tarp was the decomposing body of Aureliano Cisneros, last seen leaving a local bar with his wife. They had stormed out together as she was heard to say, "You son of a bitch, I'm going to kill you."

"On the tarp was a powdery substance that they initially thought was drugs," says Dr. Haskell, as he paces around the room, telling the story. "It wasn't." He paused for effect. "Arm and Hammer baking soda might take care of your fridge, but it doesn't do shit for the decomposing body on your front lawn."

When asked, Linda Howell said that yes, she and her husband had fought on Thursday night; but they had patched things up, and she hadn't seen him for two days, since the night of Saturday, August 6, when he had left home to go meet some friends.

When Linda Howell was arrested for the murder of her husband, law enforcement investigators had a body and a motive, but a lousy timeline.

"Are we talking twenty-four to forty-eight hours that he's been lying there?" asks Haskell. "Or are we talking four days? We have to know."

Right after bugs, Dr. Haskell loves weather. He gets a lot of both in Indiana, and that suits him just fine.

At any given time at any spot in the world certain bugs are in season. As any gardener will tell you, there are planting zones that limn the globe like meridians of longitude: In North America, for instance, Zone One is in northern Canada, Zone Ten in southern Florida. Plants that are grown in one zone may or may not be hardy in another, and spring (and all its accompaniments), as everyone knows, appears at different times in different parts of the country. You would not expect to find a honeybee busy at work in northern New York in November. In purely forensic terms, therefore, traffic deaths resulting from people swatting at bees in their cars will drop there from November until late April or May, when the incidence will again rise with the temperature.

The bugs around the body of Aureliano Cisneros were two common flies: the black blowfly and the secondary screwworm. The fly larvae—maggots—collected and preserved at the crime scene were enough evidence for Haskell to determine their species and conclude that they were in their third developmental stage, or instar, the final stage before they would crawl off to pupate and mature into adult flies.

Temperature is the key in the length of the maggots' development process: heat speeds it up, cold slows it down. And it does so on a predictable timeline that Dr. Haskell can recite like the Pledge of Allegiance. Temperature records from weather stations near Stroud were consulted for the days following the couple's argument in the bar.

"Now, we're going to need 950 to 1,150 accumulated degree hours to get blowflies to mature," he explains, "so I'm going to take the known weather data and calculate forward or backward. For her story to prove true, that he was alive and well Saturday night, the sixth, knowing that his body was discovered on the eighth, knowing that blowflies are not active at night, there's no energy adding up there. On the seventh we've got heat from sunrise on, with accumulated hours until midnight, giving us a total, maximum of 450 degree hours. Nowhere near."

Dr. Haskell continues, "You can't get the eggs hatched in those degree hours, so there is no possible way her story could be true. Sometime prior to the sixth, yes, on the fifth, we move into the ballpark for accumulated degree hours."

The death, Dr. Haskell determined, happened on Thursday night. Not long after that fact was revealed, Linda Howell accepted a plea bargain.

During the morning break, some bug school students pass around pictures of a recent group trip to the Body Farm in Tennessee. Started by legendary University of Tennessee professor William Bass, the three-acre outdoor laboratory is devoted to the study of decomposition and is the only such lab in the world. Fenced off by razor-topped barbed wire, the farm is populated with human bodies in varying stages of decay arranged in different experiments. In one, a body has been left in a car. Another body is covered with leaves. There is one uncovered on the open ground. Some are in coffins buried at varying depths, some under trees, clothed and naked, some have been embalmed and others suggest various crime scenes.

Research done at the laboratory is quoted frequently in court to aid in the understanding and interpretation of forensic evidence. After the O.J. Simpson case, for instance, Bass was called upon by the FBI to research DNA samples taken from decaying bodies. In the Simpson case, blood had been collected from the bodies of the two victims upon their discovery. Three and four days later, however, more samples were necessary, and the question arose as to whether the same amount of DNA exists in the first day's blood as in the fourth. No one could answer the question during preparation for the Simpson trial because no one had done the research.

Some people think of forensic entomology and cadaver decomposition as fringe forensic sciences. Not Dr. Haskell's bug school students, apparently. The Body Farm is a popular research site for them, as shown in the photographs that are passed around and accompanied by the kind of comments reserved in other groups for Caribbean vacations and wild game safaris.

After the break, Dr. Haskell's own slides reveal his interest in the place. So great is it, in fact, that he has willed his body to the lab, where it will be "laid out under a hickory tree, there along the river, to let nature take its course." Another slide shows his daughter Chrissy on a trip there with him, crouching next to a corpse.

The next slide displays a greatly enlarged quote from *Newsweek,* April 22, 1991. It reads: " 'Dad, You are going to have to do something with that dead cat in the freezer. It's making the milk taste funny.'—Chrissy Haskell, 9, to Neal Haskell, a forensic entomologist at Purdue University, who uses cats in his studies of maggots on corpses."

Dr. Haskell laughs like hell at one of his favorite forays into the national press.

Between his science and his demeanor, Dr. Haskell does not have a hard time getting into print. Getting into court, however, is another matter. At last count he had qualified to testify in seventeen states. But some judges simply won't have any forensic entomology in their courtrooms, and that is one of the reasons he teaches so much—more than seventy workshops so far in the United States and Canada. Neal Haskell wants nothing so much as many more people out there knocking on the court chambers, clamoring to bring maggots into court.

"Error is a big thing with the *Daubert* rule," he says. "So it's really great to have precise data. You don't want those attorneys"—he says that word in such a way that he turns it into a projectile— "telling us that they don't want bugs in the courtroom." His face sets hard, and he casts a long glance around the room and says, "You don't want someone telling you this is new science and let that defense attorney get in your face." The *Daubert* rule requires a determination of scientific reliability.

Today he is preaching to the converted. These are the men and women who hit the streets every day. There's not a potential witness for the defense among them.

To teach the students, Haskell allows them to work backward from a known time of death—something they won't often get in a real homicide—and then observe, collect and analyze. Then the students will actually raise and witness the hatching of eggs found on the carcasses. All this comes back to the pigs, who were killed at precise times and then laid out at various sites around Haskell's farm. Some are by one of two ponds, some under trees. None are near the house. It's a mini Body Farm, in fact, where all the dead are porcine.

While the students are here to learn how to provide an objective estimate of time of death, to do so they first have to become comfortable with the materials. Just how do modern investigators collect bugs?

Haskell likes to point out that the best forceps are human fingers. This usually brings a groan from somewhere in the group. Next after that are the collapsible aerial insect nets, useful for collecting fast-flying and fast-crawling adult insects. The net has an attachable handle, which increases the working distance as well as the speed the net can be manipulated. Insects that fly over the dead are strong, fast fliers, and netting them requires practice. The netting technique uses several rapid, back-and-forth, sweeping motions of the net, with reversal of the net 180 degrees on each pass. On the last pass, students are instructed to bring the open portion of the net up to chest level while rotating the opening 180 degrees, thus trapping the bugs.

The end of the net containing the insects goes directly into the wide mouth of the killing jar, where several cotton balls soaked with fresh ethyl acetate await. The killing jar is capped, and within two to five minutes the bugs will die.

Screw-cap vials await the dead specimens. Some of the vials contain 75 percent ETOH (ethyl alcohol); others are dry. If stored dry, the insects must be processed in a few hours since condensation in the vial can create excessive moisture and promote mold, which quickly damages the insects.

This process is repeated thee or four times, beginning with the aerial netting, to ensure a representative sample of all the flying insects present.

There are methods for net collection directly from the corpse, Haskell tells his students. He offers precise instructions for finger or forceps removal, complete with a reminder about the tension that should or should not be applied to hard- versus soft-carapaced insects. Following that are instructions for successful insect egg removal, since eggs must be taken back to laboratories to be hatched and raised until adulthood so that species identification can be made. Haskell keeps his nursery of bugs in his mother's basement in what he refers to as "maggot motels." In the process, he has discovered that maggots prefer to be fed beef liver.

Soil samples too must be collected from areas around the body. These are kept in two-pint (one-liter) cylindrical ice cream carton—type containers. Approximately six samples are taken from under, adjacent to and up to three feet from the body, noting the origin of each. Everything is labeled in pencil, because labels written with graphite won't be affected by preserving solutions. And some of these samples will be preserved for years. The investigator must be thinking not only about court but also about possible appeals.

Temperature readings must also be taken and recorded: ambient temperature, ground temperature, body surface temperature, maggot mass temperature, temperature at a spot where body and soil interface, and ten to twelve inches off the ground. These will be added to the mix of data. When a date of death is estimated, the temperature data for that area at that time will be requested from the National Weather Service.

The accuracy of the readings is essential because of the direct relation between hatching and temperature. And, of course, because of those defense attorneys. In the Aureliano Cisneros case, temperature readings and how they were taken became a real point of contention with one attorney.

"Oh, they tried to keep my readings out of court," recalls Haskell. "They were accurate and proper, but they were from Oklahoma City on the day of the death, not Stroud, Oklahoma. We got the hourlies and means from the east side of the city and the west side, and when it came to the cross-examination, the attorney was on me because the temps weren't from under the tarp with the body.

"The judge was a great big old cowboy, and he wasn't having any of that kind of nonsense, so he said, 'When it's hot in Oklahoma City, it's hot in Stroud.' And that was the end of it. And he admitted it."

Frequently the forensic entomologist does not see the body at the crime scene. So, the next best place for the collection of insect evidence is in the morgue. Outside and inside the body bag, in and around clothing, and in the body's cavities, the bugs will be doing or will have done their work. And it needs to be documented. Bodies found years later will retain signs of the season in which they died.

Most of the people in the bug school won't be reading the material. They will merely be collecting it after they return to their various law enforcement jobs. And so they will need to send it to a practicing forensic entomologist.

Haskell likes to tell a story about when he first started out, studying and working in economic entomology at Purdue: "We used to get bugs sent to us for identification. Mostly from farmers. All in nice little letter envelopes with return addresses. First the people would swat them, then they would take them to the post office, where they'd get cancelled. I'd open them up and there would be these little squished legs and wings. You don't want to do that."

These days he recommends several things to his students: that they don't leave specimens in hot cars for any length of time and that they try to get transport to the entomological laboratory by direct hand delivery through police agencies. Failing that, he recommends overnight mail, Federal Express or UPS, and no, he does not recommend explaining to the shipper what the package contains.

"But get them here alive," he said, urging significant packing and temperature protection.

Entomology doesn't just aid in knowing the time of death. It can also tell investigators where the death occurred. Insect species may be found in very particular places at specific times of the year in certain parts of the world. If a body is found harboring insects or insect material outside the range or season of that insect, that fact suggests the corpse was moved. That may lead investigators to a suspect living near the insect's natural habitat. The absence of insects when they should be present can be just as telling.

Insects, or more specifically, untreated insect bites, can provide evidence of abuse or neglect in both children and the elderly when detected by properly trained emergency room physicians, Haskell says.

After the morning lecture, it's lunch downtown and out to the farm to check the pigs.

There aren't a lot of services in Rensselaer, Indiana. There's one of everything, though, and that includes restaurants. There are several bars—Haskell's favorite, the City Office and Pub, included—some fast-food joints and, of course, the Busy Bee, but when someone says, "I'll meet you for dinner at the restaurant," they mean at *the* restaurant, and that is Devon's, where the helpings are enormous, the coffee is poured all day and many things are made with whole milk and cream.

After lunch, the Indiana sun cooks the day. Tonight promises one of those storms that people from the East have seen only in movies. All afternoon long, it whispers its imminence in the slow, hot and cold breeze at the farm.

Also on the breeze is the smell of death.

At 1:30 P.M., in the fry of the afternoon sun, the individual lab groups approach one dead and rotting pig at a time, everyone displaying the marked, respectful hesitancy they bring from their day jobs. Rule number one in death scene investigation: Never rush up to a body. Not only is there no reason to, but there is good reason not to. Evidence is easily trampled.

Looking at the pigs, it is easy to remember Haskell's dictum that when one biological clock stops, others begin. The place is swarming with flies. They are doing their jobs like clockwork.

There are five major stages of decomposition: fresh, bloat, decay, dry and remains. Moving from one to the next is more of a slide on a continuum than a step to a discrete stage. Along this continuum, different insects come and go, in what is known as insect succession. The different kinds of insects need to be collected to reveal where in the cycle the investigator has entered the picture and to identify a relative time on the continuum, based on insect succession. The beginning of the continuum is very accurate, but this method of telling time grows less accurate as the time from death extends. In a six-day-old case (where the body was discovered six days after the death), that can put the investigator off by plus or minus twelve hours. In a six-month-old case, the difference can be a matter of days.

There are a few thousand species of carrion insects in the United States. But the forensic entomologist must be more discerning than that, for there are ninety species of blowflies alone. Flies are the initial colonizers of and feeders on carrion. Beetles generally feed on the eggs of flies, although some beetles are carrion beetles. Fire ants, which are nasty inhabitants of the South, carry off the eggs of blowflies. They can have a major impact on the bugs and therefore on what can be read at the scene. Identifying the species, calculating air and soil temperatures and awaiting the hatching of insect eggs in the lab can be slow and arduous. Eventually, a timeline will begin to form. But it doesn't happen overnight.

But, as Haskell likes to say, "Time's fun when you're having flies."

Consider the flies alone. Within the ninety species, the investigator must identify the sex as well as the species. The females, with their keen olfactory sense, can smell death from a mile and a half away and will be the first to the scene. Identifying a female can be done by looking at her eyes: Female blowflies' eyes are widely set; the eyes of males are so close they almost touch. Species can be distinguished by examining the rows of hairs that appear on every fly. Different species, different hair—all ninety of them. There are also subtle distinguishing color, size and overall appearance variations among species. One of the bluebottle flies, *Calliphora vomitoria,* for instance, looks a lot like a B-29, in Haskell's view.

Then there are the various things that bugs can do relating to unnatural death. Cockroaches, for instance, can leave distinguishing (and to the untrained eye, confusing) tracks when traveling through a bloody crime scene. Ants can leave marks on flesh that have been mistaken for child abuse. Bees are well-known precipitants to vehicular accidents, but detecting a fatal bee sting could also be the difference in a double indemnity insurance payment, if the cause of death is ruled a heart attack. During the warm months, moths, just out minding their own business, will be collecting all over automobile license plates in the course of a driver's day. If that driver kills someone in one bug zone and then drives into another to dump the body, the evidence will be right there, ready to read. Body lice and mosquitoes, as well as maggots, may contain the DNA of a victim and, in some cases, of a perpetrator, too. They may also contain drugs used by the victim.

Dr. Haskell teaches his students to sweep the vegetation surrounding a recent death for mosquitoes. He is very clear on this: You might get lucky and pick up the perpetrator's DNA in the blood taken by the insect. And he knows it can happen, having worked a rape case that came down to DNA extracted from body lice. That kind of analysis might not make it into every court, he realizes, but having it, doing the science right and adding it to the evidence might very well dislodge a pre-trial confession from the guilty party.

After a long, hot, dirty, dusty and smelly afternoon in the sun with dead pigs, the logical thing to do, of course, is roast a hog.

Pork loin and Old Scratch beer on a warm Indiana night combine to make a convincing argument for a tour of the farm in the front cab of a pickup truck. Bumping along the eight hundred acres of Haskell's farm with a beer between the knees, the hues of twilight and the warm farm breeze thrumming on the sunflowers and sorghum, it's hard to imagine that the talk can turn to murder. But it does.

Take the case, Haskell says, of the female skeleton found in the oak and maple woodland of the Cumberland Mountains in late January. She had a hundred-cell paper wasp nest inside her skull. All but about a half dozen cells appeared empty, indicating that the nest had been occupied the year before. It appeared to have been a large and active colony of *Polistes* wasps, which begin nesting in April in that part of the country and only nest in clean, dry sites. A single sphaerocerid puparial case was also found in the cranium. But they invade a corpse only at full bloat. Counting back from the time it would have taken for the skull to be clean and dry enough to interest the wasps, and then back to the puparial state of the sphaerocerid, the estimated postmortem interval (PMI), or time from death to discovery, was set at approximately eighteen

months. Dental records identified the dead woman, who had disappeared two years before the skeleton was discovered.

An even more precise measurement involved the skeletonized
remains of a baby, recovered from a shallow grave on a narrow
ledge on the side of a crater in Hawaii. In this case, beetles solved
the crime.

Besides blowflies, a wide variety of other insects colonize dead
tissue and are attracted to a corpse in an orderly, progressive
process termed succession. The successive nature of the insects
allows the entomologist, when supplied with a representative
sample of the bugs, to develop a picture of the circumstances surrounding the death.

In the Hawaii case, which bugs showed up was less important
than which bugs did not. The absence of certain mite species
quickly shortened the original estimated PMI from seventy-six
days to slightly over fifty-two days. It later turned out that the
death had occurred in the morning fifty-three days prior to the
collection of the remains.

More than five hundred other cases have been brought to
Haskell, making him the man people think of when they think of
bugs on the dead. Of course, there are other well-known expert
forensic entomologists in the world. Wayne Lord, the FBI's
medicocriminal entomologist, is known as "Lord of the Flies," but
Haskell is considered to be, in the field of justice, more like one of
us, Mr. Everyman, down in the soil, just getting his hands dirty in
search of the truth.

Sometimes Dr. Haskell takes his show on the road, teaching
cops at clinics far from his Hoosier home. These days, though, he
does it without the transport of his trusty and recognizable mini-
van with the custom plates. It sits parked at home with almost
200,000 miles on the odometer. For out-of-state trips now, he
travels in rental cars. Flying is out of the question: too much stuff
to take along, way too many questions to answer at security gates.

How would you explain, for instance, the maggot hotels, complete with slivers of fresh liver? Or, for quick courses, the prekilled baby pigs laid out in the large, snap-topped Rubbermaid containers? It's just not worth the aggravation.

And so, on any given day, Haskell can be found crisscrossing America's heartland in a rented American sedan, with his portable bug school neatly tucked in the trunk, as he munches from jumbo bags of Jay's potato chips and listens to Tom Clancy books on tape, occasionally pulling over to read a chapter or two of books like *Panzer Commander* or to visit a World War II scout car dealer in Akron, Ohio, where he might pick up another vintage military vehicle. He currently owns nine.

"I convinced my wife and my mother that tinkering with the big toys keeps down my stress level," he says with a raise of an eyebrow and a laugh.

Both women are soft-spoken, attentive and intelligent women of great character and perception. They merely smile at any suggestion that he could ever put anything over on either of them. And both of them are in the business, in their own fashion. Haskell's mother has grown accustomed to hearing her son enter the lab in her basement at all hours of the day or night, when an insect must be preserved or a colony must be examined. She has learned to tune out the sounds of what others might consider to be some of the strangest experiments in law enforcement going on beneath her kitchen.

Jane Haskell, the scientist's wife, is a trusted and keen lab technician and processor of the bugs of the world. Both women accept his antics. And anyway, what's a few military vehicles in a family, if it keeps him down on the farm?

When it's time to leave the Haskell farm, with the slaughtered hogs still providing data for eager students of the insect detective, the drive in any direction goes right through the heart of America. You don't have to stand back in this part of the country to get a perspective on the place; it's right under your nose. Everywhere there are solid homes making up a community whose pride is well-founded. At the edges of one end of town are the car dealerships, bearing the names of their owners. In another direction, heading out past Bazz's roller rink, the town shakes out to its last few houses and then softly returns to soil.

Chances are good that by the end of the day, Dr. Neal Haskell's phone will ring, and he'll pack up his nets, boxes, Rubbermaid containers and books on tape and head out on these roads, in search of a few good bugs.

Eight

EXHUMATION

My mother was born in Russian Poland in 1901. Years later she would tell her children that Tsar Nicholas II would "wake up on the wrong side of the bed some mornings" and order a pogrom. Then the Cossacks would gallop through the Jewish village in which her father was the rabbi, randomly killing anyone they happened to see. Many times during my childhood, my mother would recount for us how she and her sister hid from the marauding troops in the septic hole, amid the human waste, to avoid being killed. Later, she survived the slaughters of World War I.

She immigrated to America in the early 1920s, following her older brother Jake, who also fled the pogroms. They were two of sixteen children in her family; the other fourteen chose to stay behind in the country that was their home. She had been a dental student at a university in Poland. In New York City she became a sewing machine operator in a dress factory in Manhattan's West Side garment district. There was no weekly salary; she was paid by the piece. She was very fast and therefore was able to save enough money by 1930 to sail back and visit her family. On that trip she met my father. Though she couldn't convince any of her siblings to come back with her, she returned to America with a husband. They soon started a family.

Then the world went into chaos with the rise of Hitler and the Second World War. My mother spent the rest of her life regretting that she had been unable to convince any more of her family to move to America. They all were eventually swept up in the hatred of anti-Semitism and taken away to a concentration camp. All fourteen of her European siblings were killed in Auschwitz.

It was with a particular and deeply personal poignancy, then, that years later I found myself on an airplane one night, flying off to Siberia to examine exhumed remains thought to be those of the Romanov family. I was particularly mindful of my childhood thoughts about Tsar Nicholas II, whom I grew up hating. I sat up that night on the long flight with Dr. Lowell Levine, who is also Jewish, and we spoke about the irony of our traveling to Russia to identify the tsar who had so persecuted the Jews. As Lowell and I talked, I realized that along with the feelings I had inherited from my mother about Nicholas, I also felt a sense of gratitude: If not for him, she would not have left Russia and would almost certainly have died in Auschwitz.

People ask me about the effect of forensic pathology on my beliefs—year after year, body after body—and I sometimes find myself saying that I am an atheist. It is hard for me to believe in a God who would not only tolerate Hitler but also allow people to do the horrible things they do to one another. Seeing what human beings do to one another every single day for more than forty years, I have turned away from religion and toward science.

At times such as this flight to Siberia, however, I am frequently reminded that a mixture of feelings is present in most things. In this case, declaring myself an atheist is too simple. All of us in the field bring ourselves to the table when we work. And in that, we also bring our personal history, which, of course, includes our beliefs.

In the Jewish tradition we have what is known as Kaddish, the Hebrew word for a liturgical prayer. Also called the Mourner's Kaddish, one form of it is said for the dead at regular intervals during the time of grieving and reflection. And as I think about my work, I realize that I bring the Kaddish along with my science each time I go to work, and that these are my offerings for the dead.

In 1979, a filmmaker for the Russian Interior Ministry named Gely Ryabov uncovered a pile of charred gray bones buried beneath a layer of old wooden train tracks. He had been looking for those particular bones for a long time: Some might say it had become his obsession. But despite his intense interest, Ryabov kept this discovery secret for a decade. Fears that the Soviet government would secretly destroy what he had found kept him silent until perestroika and the promises it brought of more openness and fairness toward his discovery. During that intervening decade, DNA analysis had been developed.

The story of the bones began during World War I, when Lenin and the Bolsheviks forced the abdication of Tsar Nicholas II, the last in an unbroken line of Romanovs, the royal family who had ruled Russia for three hundred years since Peter the Great. The tsar's family was held hostage in a house in Ekaterinburg, Siberia. A series of events pitted the forces of Lenin, the Bolsheviks and the Red Army against assorted anarchists, ethnic groups and monarchists, the last of whom supported the royal family.

On the night of July 16, 1918, the Romanov family was awaiting evacuation. The party consisted of Tsar Nicholas II; his wife, the tsarina of Russia, Alexandra Feodorovna; their four daughters, Olga, Tatiana, Marie and Anastasia; the youngest, their son, Alexis, who was a hemophiliac and was attended by a personal physician; and three domestic servants.

At about midnight, as the White Russian army was approaching to free the Romanovs from the Reds, the group was summoned to the basement of the house where they were being held. On the order of Lenin, they were shot, bayoneted and beaten.

The corpses were loaded into a truck and driven to an abandoned mine shaft, where they were stripped. Then an attempt was made to burn the bodies using gasoline, which, the assassins soon discovered, was impossible. Gasoline, which burns at about 1,500 degrees Fahrenheit, does not burn sufficiently hot to cremate a body. Cremation requires about 2,800 degrees Fahrenheit for thirty minutes. Interestingly, Hitler's followers made the same mistake decades later when they tried unsuccessfully to cremate him as he had requested.

The bodies were then dumped into the mine shaft and acid was thrown on them. The following night, after it became apparent that too many people knew of the corpses' whereabouts, they were removed to another site, where a large hole had been dug beneath abandoned railroad tracks. After repeated attempts, the two smallest bodies were partially burned and the charred fragments left in the mine shaft. The others were buried a few miles away at the railroad site.

Another strand of this story began to develop in 1920, when following a suicide attempt in Berlin, a young woman began to make some startling claims. Through a fog of what she maintained was amnesia, she claimed to be the tsar's youngest daughter, Anastasia. She stuck to her story until her death in 1984, in Charlottesville, Virginia, where she died under the name Anna Anderson.

In 1992, I was part of a team invited to Russia by the U.S. State Department and the Russian government to assist in the identification of the bones found by Gely Ryabov and geologist Alexander

Avdonin. It was an historic undertaking. Since their disappearance, the mystery of the Romanovs' fate had puzzled the world. Led by forensic anthropologist Dr. William Maples, our group included my colleague, Dr. Lowell Levine, and Cathryn Oakes, a hair and fiber expert who later married Dr. Levine.

Although eleven people had reportedly been executed on that fateful night in Ekaterinburg, the remains of only nine bodies were retrieved from the burial site. All of those bodies were completely skeletonized except one, which we identified as that of the physician. Some of his abdominal tissues were still present and had turned into the soaplike decomposition product known as adipocere, or "grave wax," which is caused by the hardening of human fat that has come into contact with water. Adipocere can resist decay for decades.

We found two World War I bullets preserved in that adipocere, thereby dating the death and ruling out, for instance, that this body might have been among the many later casualties of Stalin's purges.

Since the bodies were skeletonized, Dr. Maples's expertise and marvelous skill as a forensic anthropologist were crucial in identifying which bones belonged to which body, as well as in determining the age, sex, race and height of the decedent.

Dr. Levine's odontology was particularly important in the identification of Alexandra, whose unusually fine dental work was available only in Germany at that time. She had often traveled there to visit her family.

Two bodies were not found. The Russians believed the missing bodies to be those of Marie and Alexis, but we found that they were Alexis and Anastasia.

Of course, it is more romantic to think of Anastasia out there in the world, brought up, as the fairy tale suggests, by a good hunter in the forest who, when ordered to kill the child and bring the evil king her heart, instead brings him the heart of a deer. But it didn't happen like that in real life. When Lenin ordered people killed, they were killed.

Our findings were confirmed, for us at least, by the hair of a (royal) head.

Before her marriage, Tsarina Alexandra had been the Princess Alix of Hesse and the Rhine. She was the granddaughter of England's Queen Victoria, whose line extends through females to Prince Philip, the husband of England's current queen, Elizabeth. To assist in the identification of the disinterred bones, the prince gave blood and hair samples. That permitted conclusive comparisons of his mitochondrial DNA with that extracted from the skeletal remains of Alexandra and her children.

Hair samples plucked from the scalp tell us even more than those cut from the head. Plucked hairs include a root bulb containing cells with nuclei, which contain two strands of DNA—one from each parent. This standard type of DNA is known as nuclear or genomic DNA.

Mitochondrial DNA is present in the cytoplasm of the cell and is more abundant and more stable than nuclear DNA. The shaft of the hair contains abundant mitochondrial DNA, which is inherited only from our mothers; all the children of the same mother carry the same mitochondrial DNA. It can also be found in our bones, even after hundreds of years. Cremation, however, will destroy it, as it will nuclear DNA.

Nuclear DNA is present in the head of the sperm. Mitochondrial DNA is present in the tail. At conception, the head of the sperm enters the egg and unites with the nucleus of the ovum to form a zygote. During entry, the tail of the sperm falls off, losing the father's mitochondrial DNA and leaving only that of the mother in the fertilized cell.

For forensic purposes, that same mitochondrial DNA can be retrieved in hairs found in brushes, combs or even shower drains. But, as mentioned, it won't allow us to distinguish between siblings.

To confirm the identity of the skeleton tentatively identified by anthropological measurements as Tsar Nicholas, we matched his

DNA with DNA from his brother's remains, which were disinterred from the Romanov burial site in St. Petersburg.

And Anna Anderson? Was she Anastasia, as she claimed? By this time she was dead and had been cremated, thereby precluding any DNA testing. But it was discovered that tissue samples had been retained by a hospital in Germany where she had had an operation decades before. DNA technology is so strong and marvelous that we can now take a microscopic slide, lift off the cover slip and retrieve enough DNA from that slide to make an identification. And this is what was done for Anna Anderson with a tissue slide from her old operation.

The DNA from the samples was compared with the Romanov bone sample and Prince Philip's DNA. It did not match.

So who was she?

As early as 1927—seven years after her original claims of royalty—a private investigator had maintained that she was, in fact, Franzisca Schanzkowska, a Polish peasant who had vanished just days before "Anastasia" was rescued from a canal in Berlin. In an effort to gain closure on this issue, a maternal grandnephew of the missing peasant woman was located in Germany, and he provided a blood test for DNA comparison. It was a positive match. Anna Anderson was not Anastasia.

The remains of Anastasia and Alexis were never found.

> Dante Gabriel Rossetti
> Buried all of his libretti
> Thought the matter over then
> And dug them all back up again.
> — ANONYMOUS

What this little rhyme fails to mention is that when the fine Pre-Raphaelite painter and poet buried his verses, he did so along with the body of Elizabeth Siddal, his beloved wife and model. She committed suicide in 1862 by taking an overdose of laudanum, a tincture of opium, following a long period of melancholy and tuberculosis. In his grief and guilt, Rossetti buried a manuscript of his poems with his wife. Some years later he had her body exhumed, and the poems were recovered. It seems he had subsequently become convinced that his work was of greater value than he had previously believed.

Rossetti is not alone among the greats of literature whose lives—or deaths—have involved exhumation. Several times in history, groups have gathered to push for the exhumation of no less than William Shakespeare, whose eulogists, according to some, tossed their funereal speeches into the grave of the Bard. Those manuscripts would have been printed on rag paper and may, in fact, have survived to date. If they have, they are of inestimable value.

Then, of course, there is the ridiculous debate over who Shakespeare actually was, and whether, in fact, the author was really Francis Bacon; Edward de Vere, the seventeenth Earl of Oxford; or Christopher Marlowe. This inanity continues to motivate some to call for exhumations of all involved. In fact, for a long time, Marlowe's original manuscripts were thought to be buried with his great friend Sir Thomas Walsingham, whose tomb was subsequently opened in 1956. No manuscripts were found.

And, finally, there is the question of whether Shakespeare was poisoned by a son-in-law whom he had written out of his will soon before his death. But don't get the exhumation people started on that one. All this discussion is of great interest to those whose careers, for better or for worse, are closely associated with the work they've done disinterring the dead.

One of these is Jim Starrs, known in some circles as "Bone Hunter." Starrs, a professor of law and forensic science at George Washington University, is currently involved with a project that has resulted in the exhumation of several descendants of the brothers of George Washington.

In 1995 Starrs was involved in the exhumation of legendary

outlaw Jesse James to determine whether the correct man was buried under that name. (He was.) Starrs also wants to dig up Meriwether Lewis, but to date his requests to do so have been rejected by the National Park Service, which owns the land where he is buried. Lewis died under what some consider mysterious circumstances in a Tennessee tavern in 1809. History has listed Lewis as a suicide, but Starrs believes he was murdered, as do at least 160 of Lewis's descendants, who signed a statement supporting the exhumation.

The questions to be answered in George Washington's case concern whether the father of our country—or perhaps one of his relatives—also fathered a son named West Ford, with Venus, a young slave who lived on the estate of his brother John Augustine Washington.

George and Martha Washington had no children together. Because Martha bore four children in her first marriage, the suggestion was made long ago that our first president was sterile. Comparison of a Y chromosome inherited from one of his brothers with that of a West Ford descendant could indicate whether a Washington family member was Ford's father. But it could not prove that George Washington was the father.

Hair samples believed to be from the president exist, but according to the Mount Vernon Ladies Association, the FBI has analyzed samples of hair identified as Washington's from Mount Vernon and four other museums and failed to recover enough DNA even to determine whether they were from the same person.

The case reminds us, of course, of that of Sally Hemings, the slave who was the longtime companion of Thomas Jefferson. Most historians had long dismissed the stories of sexual trysts between Jefferson and Hemings until 1998, when DNA evidence supported the long-held belief of her descendants that America's third president fathered her family.

The question remains—will George Washington eventually be disinterred? Exhuming presidents, after all, is not without prece-

dent. The body of Zachary Taylor was exhumed in 1991 from his
family crypt in Louisville, Kentucky, after a Florida author raised
the question of arsenic poisoning of the man known as "Old
Rough and Ready" and suggested that Taylor had been murdered
because of his opposition to the spread of slavery to the Southwest.
Had he been murdered, he would take the place of Abraham Lincoln as the first slain American president. Taylor's body had been
in the ground for 141 years before it was disinterred. After examination of his bones, teeth, hair and nails, no sign of arsenic poisoning was found.

Just how far does justice extend? If an author can cast enough
doubt on the cause and manner of a president's death to warrant
disrupting the sanctity of the tomb, should the same method be
used to establish paternity?

It has certainly been done to other men.

In March 1998, the world's attention returned to actor and
singer Yves Montand, who had died in 1991. At that time he had
been involved in a paternity battle being waged in Paris by a
young woman who claimed to be his daughter. Although Montand's family was said to be revolted by the court decision that
ordered the exhumation, the DNA tests confirmed their belief
that he was not the woman's father.

Should we exhume presidents for this reason, as well?

No, according to the anti-exhumation people, who, for a variety of reasons, steadfastly refuse to accept that anything should
necessitate disturbing a body's eternal rest. Most of us may shud-
der at the idea of exhuming someone for plain curiosity, profit or
career enhancement, but we know that at times the need for truth
outweighs objections to disturbing a grave.

That was certainly the prevailing feeling in our nation's capital
in 1998, when, with appropriate solemnity and protocol, the
remains of a twenty-four-year-old fighter pilot were removed from
the Tomb of the Unknowns. He is unknown no more. Science has
given him back his name, and the family of Michael J. Blassie

knows his fate and was able to bury him with the recognition he deserved.

The future of the Tomb of the Unknowns is less certain: Should the remains of another unknown soldier be placed under the inscription HERE RESTS IN HONORED GLORY AN AMERICAN SOL-DIER-KNOWN BUT TO GOD? Today, DNA technology applied to bone, tissues and hair leaves few, if any, dead persons unknown. So why shouldn't we seek to solve these unanswered questions by opening graves once considered eternal? The answer depends largely on our feelings about exhumation.

Unsealing the Tomb of the Unknowns at Arlington National Cemetery required the use of a diamond-tipped blade applied for twelve hours to slice through the ten inches of granite slabs. Clearly, at one time, we believed that the unknown's remains— including in this case a pelvis, right upper arm and four ribs— would never be disturbed.

In fact, at the ceremony prior to exhuming Michael Blassie's remains, Defense Secretary William Cohen said, "We disturb this hallowed ground with profound reluctance." The reluctance we feel seems, in this case, to have been outweighed by the family's demand for the truth.

American courts are reluctant to order an exhumation when the next of kin objects—as when the judge denied the Massachusetts prosecutors' request to exhume the body of Mary Jo Kopechne, the passenger in Senator Edward Kennedy's car when it plunged off a bridge on Chappaquiddick Island. The prosecutor wanted to establish the precise cause of death: specifically, whether she drowned or died of blunt injuries on impact. But her parents objected to the exhumation, and none was performed. In that case, the state could have ordered an autopsy before the burial, but didn't. Once a body is interred, the common law doctrine of the Sanctity of the Sepulchre gives greater weight to the right of the family to prevent disturbing the dead.

What we might learn from a body is never known to us until

we start to look. We might find a button clenched in its hands or a killer's preserved footprint underneath it. Trace evidence in illicit burials frequently reveals flora or soil from the scene where the murder took place that traveled with the body to the burial site.

Exhumation is a painstaking process that begins with the very ground in which the person is buried. Soil samples are taken to ensure that elements in the earth, such as arsenic, can be identified, so that any minerals seeping into the body are not mistaken for a cause of death.

This is an important first step. In a memorable case in London at the beginning of the last century, a man who had buried several wives was executed for their murders—although he maintained his innocence—after they were exhumed and all found to contain high levels of arsenic. Years later, an enterprising student tested the soil around the coffins of the reinterred women and found arsenic—no surprise, since it is one of the most abundant of the heavy metals. The man may have simply outlived his wives only to be hanged for it.

Preventing inaccuracies is essential to the success of exhumation, of course. Such prevention begins with efficiency. I don't like to have bodies out of the ground for long. In fact, it is always my intention to return a body to the grave the same day we remove it. There are exceptions of course, but the rule is to be as quick yet as thorough as you can be, with a minimal amount of disruption to the grave.

But when I say this to people, they frequently think we move into the cemetery with ground penetrating radar devices. We don't, except in cases of ancient graves or illicit burials. Ground penetrating radar (GPR)—also known as ground piercing radar or subsurface interfering radar—can also be helpful in locating mass graves. It was used in Kosovo, for instance.

The technology is much like that of a very powerful metal detector. The other principle at work is the same as that of speed traps, where radar is bounced off an object and sends back an impression.

We use the same equipment in cemetery exhumations that is used by that cemetery to bury bodies. These days that includes a backhoe as well as grave diggers.

Exhumations are typically scheduled for 7 A.M., hours before the regular daily business of the cemetery will be conducted. We begin by locating the grave. Often that is not as easy as it sounds.

Cemeteries appear to consist of neat rows outlined in head-stones, but that is not the picture you get once you go under-ground. Caskets drift. Sometimes family plots contain many graves under one communal headstone. As a result, 5 percent of the time that we go into the ground, we initially find the wrong body.

All cemeteries have maps of where bodies are supposed to be. After we consult the map and determine where to dig, the ceme-tery staff moves in with six-foot-long poles to stick into the ground in search of the casket or casket liner. When the casket is located, the backhoe moves in.

About thirty years ago, people stopped putting caskets directly into the ground. For several reasons, we now use cement liners, complete with a concrete top, into which the casket is placed. If you take a walk through an old cemetery you will notice sagging in the grave sites. This is a result of collapsed coffins. This was upsetting to the mourners as well as to the people who have to mow the grass. Also, the cement liners are sealed with an adhesive designed to make them watertight. Usually, though, the adhesive doesn't hold over time, and when water gets in, it can't get out. In this aspect of my work, water is a real problem.

As the disinterment continues, chains will remove the cement liner top, and straps will be placed under the coffin. It will be lifted out and transported by hearse to wherever the autopsy will be performed. This may be the office of the local medical examiner, the local hospital morgue, if it is a criminal case, or a local funeral home, as in most civil cases.

The moment before the casket is opened is just what you think it would be: very exciting and very troubling. I always have the same questions: What will I find? Will it be the right body? How intact will the remains be?

Before the exhumation I will have made provisions to ensure positive identification: I'll have the dental records, the medical history, and any records on file with the funeral home or from the family of objects known to have been buried with the deceased. The things that are placed into coffins run the gamut.

Family members may or may not be present at the disinterment. They certainly will not be present for the examination, though they may be needed for identification. I usually have close phone contact with at least one family member before and right after the procedure. This person may be waiting at a nearby hotel.

One of the most remarkable exhumation cases I have ever handled included one of the most poignant family moments I have ever witnessed.

On June 12, 1963, Medgar Evers was shot in the back while leaving his car at his family home in Jackson, Mississippi. He was thirty-three years old, a civil rights leader and a prominent official in the Mississippi NAACP, in charge of voter registration.

The bullet that struck him entered his right back, went through a lung, exited his body through his right chest, traveled through a window in his house and finally struck the refrigerator. Barely alive, he was taken by ambulance to the nearby University of Mississippi Hospital, where his personal physician, Dr. Albert Britton, was initially prevented from providing emergency treatment because Dr. Britton was black.

Investigators at the scene recovered the rifle that had fired the bullet. It was found in some bushes about a hundred yards away from the Evers house. The rifle was traced back to a man named Byron De La Beckwith, and it retained his palm print.

EXHUMATION

The attorney general at the time vigorously pursued the prosecution of Beckwith and brought the case to trial twice, both times resulting in hung juries.

Almost thirty years later Dr. Lowell Levine and I were invited to lecture to the Mississippi District Attorneys' Association at its annual meeting in Biloxi. Over dinner, Bobby DeLaughter, an assistant district attorney, and Ed Peters, his boss, brought us up to date on the Evers case. Peters, the Jackson district attorney, was considering reopening the case. But in the course of doing some investigating they had discovered that the autopsy report, the rifle and the fatal bullet were missing. Specifically, they needed to determine the cause of death, and they wanted me to tell them if, without the original autopsy report, it could be established.

You never ask a medical examiner whether you need an autopsy or an exhumation: It's like asking a barber whether you need a haircut. I told them that even after all these years there should be enough skeletal remains present to reconstruct the gunshot wound if the bullet had struck bone on its way in or out. I told them that the bone would reveal the bullet's trajectory, which is what a prosecutor would need in order to show the jury the cause of death.

In the meantime, Bobby DeLaughter, the assistant district attorney assigned to the case, found the missing rifle in the home of his ex-wife, whose father had been the judge in both trials in the 1960s. DeLaughter had remembered that his father-in-law had had a rifle collection, which he had passed on to his daughter when he died, and when DeLaughter went to look, sure enough, the Medgar Evers rifle was there.

People think only serial murderers take trophies. When I was investigating the death of Martin Luther King, Jr., for the U.S. Congress, there were some important X rays we wanted to get from Harlem Hospital that had been taken when King had been stabbed in New York City years before. They were missing. It happens all the time; people take X rays, brain tissue, microscopic slides—almost anything—as collectibles.

So, the Evers rifle was found. But not the bullet.

In order to exhume, I knew we would need permission from the next of kin. But Evers had served his country in war and was buried in Arlington National Cemetery. I knew from experience that exhumations of such a prominent person sometimes created perception problems with the public. So I urged the prosecutor to get permission from all the pertinent relatives, so that there could be no questions later on. He got permission from all three children, as well as from Myrlie Evers, the widow.

One of the children, Van, would give his permission only if he could be present at the disinterment and the autopsy. At the time of the exhumation, Van was about the same age his father had been when he died. He had no memory of his dad. Van traveled to Arlington, then traveled by hearse with the casket to Albany, New York, where I was to perform the autopsy.

The arrival of the casket caused quite a stir. It had been shipped in a pine transportation crate that by chance had been manufactured in Memphis, and when one of the morgue men saw that it had come from Memphis, he called the *Times Union*, Albany's paper. Speculation quickly spread that we were performing an autopsy on Elvis Presley. Suddenly there was worldwide attention on what we were doing.

When we opened the casket, we were all shocked to find that Medgar Evers looked as though he had died only the day before. His hands lay in repose over his abdomen; pine needles that had been placed in the coffin with him were still green. His Masonic pin, hat and apron were present and intact. My immediate thought was to call Van right over, instead of waiting until after the autopsy to let him view his dad. He was at a nearby hotel.

We draped the casket with some blankets to make it look more the way it would in a funeral parlor. Van came in, and in what remains one of the most poignant moments of my life, saw the young face of his father, of whom he had no recollection. He and Bobby DeLaughter hugged each other.

After Van left, we did what we normally do in an exhumation and autopsy, including X rays, photographs and a full examination.

We clearly saw evidence of the previous autopsy, including the Y-shaped incision as well as the incision from ear to ear at the back of the head.

We saw both the entrance and exit wounds of the bullet and were able to photograph them and reestablish the bullet trajectory, which, after all, was the main reason for the exhumation. But the X rays proved most critical to the case. They showed fragments of the bullet that had broken off when it struck the fifth rib on the way out of the body. In fact, the X rays showed a wide area of small fragments.

I knew from the prior testimony, including the 1963 ballistics report, that the bullet was a soft-nosed .30-06. Bullets like this have a lead tip instead of a full metal jacket. They are used in hunting big animals because when the soft-nosed bullet strikes, it does a lot more damage than a full metal jacket: The soft nose breaks off and leaves a lot of fragments behind. A rifle such as the one traced back to Beckwith would have put a lot of energy behind a bullet, resulting in a high-speed trajectory. The higher the speed of the bullet striking the rib, the finer the fragmentation. What we found in the Evers case is referred to as the starry sky effect, with lots of tiny little dots showing on the X ray, typical for such a rifle and such a bullet. The more fragments, the more damage to the body. While inside the body I was able to locate and remove those metal fragments.

In the end, there was enough information on the cause of death to allow the DA to proceed with a reindictment against Byron De La Beckwith and bring him to trial. It took an extradition that Beckwith fought—and finally lost—but in 1994, he went to trial in Jackson, Mississippi, for a crime he thought he had gotten away with thirty years before.

On the stand, the DA handed me the photos I had taken at the

Evers autopsy. I reviewed them for the jury. Then the jury was allowed to view them, and that put a face to the case. This can happen with an exhumation, bringing power and immediacy to a case previously made up of old testimony and ancient headlines.

The DA also handed me the test tube that held the bullet fragments I had taken from Evers at the autopsy. These too were passed to the jury, some of whom shook them gently as I had done on the stand. The sound of those little fragments beating against the glass made the bullet very real.

After the trial, some of the jurors were heard to say that the bullet fragments and autopsy photos had made Evers a real person for them and not just an historical figure. Perhaps that is why Byron De La Beckwith was finally convicted of murdering Medgar Evers. While serving a life sentence in prison, Beckwith died in early 2001 of natural causes.

The very nature of an exhumation is to revisit questions that were literally laid to rest. And sometimes when we do that, we raise more questions than we can answer. That is certainly what has happened with the case of the Boston Strangler.

Eleven women were strangled in Boston between June 1962 and January 1964. In 1967, Albert DeSalvo confessed to all eleven killings but was never charged in them. He was killed in prison in 1973 while serving a sentence on an unrelated rape conviction.

The last alleged victim of the Boston Strangler was Mary Sullivan. Her family has never believed that DeSalvo was her killer. Neither has DeSalvo's family. No physical evidence tied him to the crimes. The two families are among those who believe that the details in DeSalvo's confession were garnered from the press coverage at the time. For more than thirty years they had pressed authorities in Massachusetts to grant access to records and evidence found at the scene of Sullivan's death.

It is known that the police collected evidence from that scene, including a semen-stained bedsheet, cigarette butts and the clothes Sullivan was wearing the night she was killed. The cigarette butts are of particular interest since Sullivan did not smoke and since they are rich in DNA material. This is because the buccal cells, from the inner lining of the mouth, are a rich source of DNA. By comparison, blood samples are far less rich, since 99.9 percent of the cells in any sample are red blood cells, which contain no nuclei—and therefore no nuclear DNA. The DNA obtained from blood comes from the white blood cells, which comprise less than one thousandth of 1 percent of the cells in the blood. These days, many labs and police officers prefer to take buccal swabs when obtaining DNA samples: They are less invasive than blood tests and have a higher yield of DNA.

For years the families were met with only repeated refusals and total opposition. Sullivan's nephew and DeSalvo's brother eventually sued the office of the Commonwealth Attorney General, the Massachusetts State Police, the Boston Police and the medical examiner. Then, finally, they went to exhumation specialist Jim Starrs, who, despite the enormous opposition, was able to arrange the exhumation.

The actual exhumation and autopsy would have to be done by a forensic pathologist who could ensure the removal of anything from the body that might be of evidentiary value or that might be usable in DNA studies.

So it was at 8:15 A.M. on October 14, 2000, that I found myself in Hyannis, Massachusetts, with about thirty other people, ready to exhume the body of Mary Sullivan. By and large, all involved were volunteering their services, including Starrs, Henry Lee and me. We often perform this kind of work pro bono since it is a service for the common good.

Everything we did was videotaped, an option that had been unavailable early in my career. We wanted proper legal documentation so that no one could suggest the evidence had been altered and challenge our findings.

By 10 A.M. we were at the same funeral parlor at which Mary Sullivan had been prepared for burial thirty-six years before. As her family waited outside, we began the autopsy.

The forensic odontologist was able to identify the body through her dental records. A forensic anthropologist confirmed that her skeletal structure was that of a twenty-year-old white female. I observed that the previous autopsy incision in the first report matched with what I was seeing. We took X rays, collected hair samples and scanned the body under various light sources for any remaining trace evidence.

Then I went inside.

When Albert DeSalvo confessed to killing Mary Sullivan, he said he struck her in the head to knock her out, then strangled her. But the exhumation widened the mystery of the Boston Strangler, for I found no skull fractures or other evidence of any significant head injury. Apparently, she had been strangled.

The questions about the Boston Strangler may remain unanswered for years. One thing is for certain: The exhumation caused the prosecutors to reopen the case and to examine the original retained evidence. This has made two families happier than they have been for a very long time.

Of course, there is no guarantee that an exhumation will please anyone: Despite the determination of a family, the interests of society and the application of technology to see justice done, some exhumations simply don't turn out as they should. That certainly was the case with Willie Edwards.

On a January night in 1957, Willie Edwards disappeared in Montgomery, Alabama, leaving behind a pregnant wife and two small children. In April of that year, two fishermen working the waters of the Alabama River noticed a man's decomposed body lodged in the branches of a tree off the riverbank. Apparently the body had traveled downstream on the high waters of late winter and early spring. As the waters receded, they left behind the evidence of a terrible crime.

What we know is that on that January night in 1957, Willie Edwards was living in a place of racial unrest. Only three weeks into the new year, Alabama had already witnessed the bombings of four black churches and the dynamiting of two houses. The Ku Klux Klan was thriving, and on that night they had planned to avenge a rumor that a black Winn-Dixie deliveryman had harassed a white woman the day before.

Willie Edwards had already finished his day shift delivering for the grocery store chain but had been called back in to cover for the night driver.

In 1976, Raymond C. Britt, a self-proclaimed Klansman, obtained immunity from prosecution by giving an affidavit in which he confessed to participating in Willie Edwards's murder. He stated that on the night of January 23, 1957, he and three other men forced Willie Edwards to jump off the Tyler-Goodwin Bridge into the Alabama River.

According to the affidavit, after driving around town, the four men had located the Winn-Dixie truck with a black driver parked on a road. The driver was filling out his logbook. They ordered the man out of the truck and into their car and then proceeded to the Tyler-Goodwin Bridge. During the trip, the Winn-Dixie driver "was shoved around and slapped" while they questioned him about harassing a white woman. He sobbed and begged for his life, stating that he had not done any of the things they were questioning him about and that he had not worked on the day in question.

When they arrived at the bridge, the man was ordered out of the car and told to "hit the water." He climbed up on the bridge's railing, fifty feet above the river. He jumped.

At the time of the death, Alabama was one of two states in the country that allowed nonphysicians to autopsy the dead. The local medical examiner, Vann Pruitt, was not a doctor. No X rays were taken. After almost three months in the water, the body was badly decomposed. Pruitt wrote "undetermined" under both cause and manner of death. No one was charged.

In 1976, prosecutors tried to revive the homicide investigation. That was when I got a call from the FBI. At the time, I was the deputy chief medical examiner of New York City. The agent on the phone wanted to know whether, after twenty years, a determination of the cause and manner of death could be made in the case of a person allegedly thrown off a bridge.

I said it was possible. But I never heard back from the FBI.

Only some years later did I learn what had happened. An indictment had been brought against the three men named by Britt, the state's informant. But when the case got to court, the judge cited the death certificate's finding of "undetermined" and dismissed the case: No finding of homicide, no case, he ruled. Again, no one was charged.

Then, in 1997, I received a letter from Malinda Edwards, who had seen me discussing the death of Medgar Evers on the HBO series *Autopsy,* which I host. This television show explores how crimes are solved through forensic science. She wrote that she was the daughter of a man whom she was convinced had been murdered, but that authorities had never brought her father's killers to justice.

I called Malinda Edwards, and as we spoke I suddenly realized that this was the same case I had been called about more than twenty years before. She sent me her files, records and the autopsy report. After reviewing the records, I again spoke to her. I explained that the Medgar Evers case was resolved because not only was the family behind the exhumation but the local district attorney and the local medical examiner were fully supportive of a review, as well. In her father's case, whether or not the death certificate would be changed from "undetermined" to "homicide" would be up to the local medical examiner in the district in which the body was buried. Without official support, the fight to find Willie Edwards's killers would be extremely difficult.

EXHUMATION

As it turned out, not only did Ellen Brooks, the Montgomery County district attorney, express interest in pursuing this case, but Dr. James Lauridson, the Montgomery medical examiner—this time, a board-certified forensic pathologist—was very eager, as well. He proved to be a superb forensic pathologist. That support, combined with the consent of Sarah Edwards Salter, the widow, as well as Malinda's, gave us what we needed to proceed toward exhumation of the remains.

There was no cement liner protecting the coffin of Willie Edwards. The coffin was badly weathered. When we opened it, we discovered that the bones were completely skeletonized.

Present in the autopsy room were myself, Dr. Lauridson and Dr. Bill Rodriguez, anthropologist for the Armed Forces Institute of Pathology.

We reconstructed the skeletonized bones on the autopsy table. Did the skeletonized remains fit the race, height and weight of the deceased? Yes, they did.

There were no gunshot wounds and no stab wounds evident in the skeletonized remains. But we knew that the body had been found just above water after the river had fallen, and at the time it was originally found, it had been in the water—in fact, was transported by it—over the months it was missing.

The definition of drowning is a diagnosis of exclusion. Lauridson and I determined that since the body had been in water and since there was no other reason for the death, there was enough evidence to find that the cause of death was drowning.

The manner of death is always dependent on the circumstances. The determination of accident, suicide or homicide depends on the history. The history here consisted of evidence including a sworn affidavit stating that Willie Edwards was pulled out of his truck by four people against his will, brought to the bridge and either pushed or made to jump. Others claimed that Edwards voluntarily jumped off the bridge that night to escape.

We agreed that even if he had fallen while attempting to escape, the manner of death would still be homicide.

Cause of death: Drowning. Manner of death: Homicide.

I then went to the local telephone book and looked up Vann Pruitt, the signer of the first death certificate. I wanted to discuss his original findings with him. One of the things you don't want in cases like this is for someone like that to show up as a witness for the defense. I expected him to be very defensive.

I had another surprise in store: He was delighted to hear from me.

"I am so glad you called," he said. Pruitt explained that in 1957, his lack of medical training prevented him from making a diagnosis of drowning; "undetermined" was the only truthful finding he could have made.

Armed with the new death certificate, Montgomery County District Attorney Ellen Brooks went to the grand jury. She decided not to pursue any indictments by name but rather to present this as an investigation, hoping that in the process additional information might come to light. In a case this old, sometimes prosecutors do this, hoping to unearth anything more that might secure an indictment.

The Edwards family was shocked. Two of the four men suspected in the homicide were still alive—and although one of them claimed immunity as a state's witness, there was another man living and working in Montgomery who had previously been indicted in 1976 for the homicide of Willie Edwards. And now the obstacle that the judge had then cited—the previous "undetermined" manner and cause of death—was gone. Willie Edwards's death was a homicide in need of justice.

On February 16, 1999, a Montgomery County grand jury submitted its findings: "We have investigated the death of Willie Edwards, who disappeared on January 23, 1957. Edwards was murdered in Montgomery County by members and/or associates of the Ku Klux Klan."

But they brought no indictments against anyone. The prosecutor felt she lacked sufficient evidence after all this time.

Had I been requested to do an exhumation and autopsy when I was first called about the case by the FBI in 1976, I would have made the same findings that I finally did in 1997. Justice could have been served.

Nine

HEADS

If everything goes according to its natural plan, people live good, long lives, are buried or cremated and returned to land or sea or air; then nature works long and hard to decompose what is left.

Unnatural death changes all that. It stops human nature. Then forensic investigation begins, requiring that the work of Mother Nature be arrested, as well—that the natural decay process which does many things, including undermining identification, be halted.

If Mother Nature has been left too long at her work, identification of the dead may be very difficult. Sometimes identification can be made from teeth or DNA. But those require a match with a specimen on file. Good as they are, neither DNA nor dental work comes with a return address label.

Sometimes the only alternative in the search for identity is to rebuild something that looks almost lifelike. The obvious reason is for identification purposes. But we also do this because the individual's very identity—who he was, whether she was an alcoholic, a drug user, someone with mental health problems that might have led to wandering or suicide—may help reveal the cause and manner of death. It's almost as if we have to get to know someone to know how that person died.

Sometimes rebuilding an identity begins with a fragment of a tibia, a pelvis or a hand. But any investigator will tell you that it is a lot easier if there is a head.

It is scary and unsettling—even terrifying—to hold a human head.

There is no comparison between holding a head and holding a skull. I can keep a certain emotional distance from a skull; you can literally hold one at arm's length. But you don't have to; they are not upsetting. But a head in the morgue creates chaos.

In part, it is the soft tissue—the skin, hair and eyes, the ears and lips—that upset us so. These are the aspects of the face, of course, and it is in the millions of faces we see in a lifetime—coming at us up the street, looking out from magazine pictures, photographs or movie screens—that we make up our picture of humanity. And so it is natural that we attach such emotion to the head that we cringe at the very idea of seeing it in any unnatural setting.

But no emotional distance is possible when I have a head in my gloved hands. Actually, I don't wish to be disinterested; I never want to deny that it is, in fact, somebody's child's head that I hold. Even if I did, experience has taught me that there is no way to hold a head, no position in which to place it or prop it up, that does anything to diminish its emotional power. I have come to understand that the engulfing eeriness I feel when I confront a severed head is not something I can expect to get over.

The head of an adult male weighs about eleven pounds.

Although I know that, I will still weigh one when it comes in detached from the body. Severed heads are usually the result of a train or subway accident or of someone who has done the work of dismemberment in order to hide the victim's identity or the evidence of a crime.

The problem is in how to handle the head. In a purely clinical sense, a head is ungainly. There is literally no good way to examine one. When attached to the corpse a head lies still, anchored in the resting position of the body. On its own, however, the head cannot be put in a convenient position in which to study the brain.

Examining a head pushes me into direct conflict with the way I conduct an autopsy. Foremost for me is to show respect for the human body at all times. Part of doing this comes from maintaining the order in which I do things, one autopsy after the other, repeating a pattern of clinical behavior: Examine the clothes, remove the clothes, examine the skin, talk into the tape recorder, pick up the scalpel, make the incision, reflect (pull back) the skin, examine one organ at a time, time after time—nothing haphazard, nothing chaotic, nothing disrespectful.

But it is terribly difficult to place a head in a resting position that shows respect. People have to hold it in order to secure it, and that very act upsets the orderly pattern of the autopsy and destroys that sense of clinical calm we depend on. It simply makes chaos.

On the other end of the spectrum are those heads that have been exposed to the elements for a long time and may be clean down to the skull. Fiction and film fans may remember the scene in *Gorky Park* in which the partially decomposed skulls of three people killed in Moscow's park of that name were then turned over to insects to clean off the remaining bits of flesh before facial reconstruction. That works, as nature shows us, but it is too slow for actual forensic science. The most efficient method to clean a head down to the skull bones is to carefully boil and bleach it. Then the process of rebuilding all that has been stripped away can begin.

Of the 206 bones of the human body, 22 make up the head and face. Together, these bones protect the brain as well as most of the body's chief sensory organs—the eyes, ears, nose and tongue.

The human cranium, which is also known as the braincase, is formed by eight bones. These bones look like thin, curved plates and are fused together by fibrous joints called sutures. At the site of a suture, the bone surfaces have irregular areas of contact that look like serrations or wiggly ridges. These sutures provide resistance to shearing forces that might otherwise wrench apart the bones.

Fourteen bones shape the human face, most in symmetrical pairs. At the base of the skull is the occipital bone, which forms a joint with the first vertebra of the neck, called the atlas. The ancient Greeks felt that the atlas bone held up the head just as Atlas held up the earth. The atlas permits rotation and bending of the head on top of the cervical spine.

During infancy, the fontanelles, or soft spots between the skull bones, can be easily felt. These are unossified membranes that with age are gradually replaced by bone and become a complete bony union usually by the time we are in our twenties or thirties; the stages of this progression can aid in determining the age of unidentified skeletal remains.

The head is covered with skin and hair. The eyes have color. Eyebrows arch, noses flare, chins jut and ears have many different shapes and angles. So while we think of each face as being unique, the truth is that each individual aspect of the head is unique, as well. Each bone is yours alone; the shape, the thickness and the number of corrugations at the margins of the skull bones are unique to you; the root bulb of your hair carries strands of your mother's as well as your father's nuclear DNA; the shaft of your hair has abundant amounts of your mother's mitochondrial DNA; your lips have unique prints, as do your ears; and a single tooth can identify you and, perhaps, your dentist.

Many people think that it is mostly police who come across human remains and that when they do, those remains are found clean and dry, like those of a skeleton in anatomy class. In fact, it is rarely like that.

It's not cops who usually find skeletonized bodies—it's dogs, kids, hikers, mountain bikers or fishermen, stumbling upon remains long after nature has taken its toll. And by that time, few untrained people can recognize what it is they are looking at. That being the case, when an unidentified, skeletonized body is found, a forensic anthropologist may be called in to assist in recovering and removing the remains.

Once the bones are removed from the scene and taken back to the lab, they will be cleaned, reconstructed into the human form and studied to determine the trauma pathways—shots or stab wounds that splintered ribs or cracked the skull, bones broken by blunt force trauma. A biological profile will be compiled: ancestry (race), sex, age, stature and body build, and pathology and individual characteristics, such as long-healed fractures or metal prostheses.

Most questions are answered by simple observation: There are basically three races on earth, each with distinct skull and facial shapes; women have distinct circular pelves as opposed to men's, which are more triangular; the bones of the body change as we age and when disease processes develop. All of those changes allow the anthropologist to make basic determinations about the remains.

I can tell by looking at the bones whether they are animal or human. I can also tell by the extent to which the soft tissues have left the body whether it is an old or recent skeleton, and therefore whether I have to do a "tongue test" to determine age. After about a hundred years, the calcium leaves the bones. Old bones get the tongue test; if my tongue sticks, calcium is still present, meaning the bones are probably less than fifty years old and we need to call in the police to investigate.

In cases of old bones I will defer to a forensic anthropologist.

One of the main reasons for doing so is that although there are certain characteristics I can infer, these do not include racial identification. If there is any question of the bones having come from a Native-American burial ground, for instance, we want to know right away so we can protect it.

In the last few years great advances have been made in extracting mitochondrial DNA from very old bones. But what many people forget is that it is still necessary to get a tentative identification of the remains to know whom to compare them with. There is no worldwide DNA database of the dead.

In the same way, the ability to read the DNA in a bone fragment does not necessarily mean that the expensive, time-consuming science of DNA analysis needs to be used, since along the spectrum from drawing a face to analyzing DNA, there are many places to get a match.

In this way, and just about every day, the newest sciences meet some of the oldest.

It began with Paul Revere, the noted silversmith and official courier to the Continental Congress, who, along with his famous midnight ride, is well known in some circles for making the country's first postmortem dental evidence identification. He made it on Dr. Joseph Warren, a general in the Revolutionary Army who had been killed at the battle of Bunker Hill and was initially buried in a grave with another man. The desire to honor the general led to his exhumation ten months later and to Revere, who had made him a dental appliance. Revere sadly confirmed the identification.

The next high-profile use of the science came in 1849 when Dr. George Parkman, a wealthy benefactor of Harvard Medical School, was murdered by Dr. John White Webster, a professor of chemistry and mineralogy at the school. Dr. Webster was hanged for the murder after charred dental and denture fragments found in the Harvard chemistry laboratory furnace were identified by the maker of the denture as having belonged to Parkman.

For decades, the science of forensic dentistry did not change much because the mouth itself hadn't changed. It relied upon the presence or absence of teeth, on the surfaces filled, the filling material, the appliances built for and the impressions left by the mouth.

Two inventions, however, did radically change all dentistry: the X ray and the high-speed drill. They are interrelated, since the diagnostic X-ray examination of a tooth is critical to planning the treatment. A third influence, almost tangential, was the growth of insurance carriers, whose demand for verification of the need for treatment has generated untold millions of X rays. In forensic circles these X rays are considered a vast pool of evidence.

The science of forensic dentistry is one of pattern recognition. Much like fingerprints and tire prints, blood spatters and tool marks, teeth leave patterns or impressions, whether it be in the goop you clench at your dentist's office to make an appliance, the chewing gum you leave in an ashtray, a drinking straw you nervously nibble and discard or the skin of someone you bite. They are different kinds of impressions, of course, but comparable.

For instance, a comparison can be made by a forensic odontologist from a photograph of the bruises left on someone else's skin to either the bite mark impression on file with your dentist, or to a court-ordered dental impression a defendant may be required to provide.

Your dentist does much the same work as those dentists who work with the dead—except the latter are called forensic odontologists (odontology being the Greek name inherited from Europe, and one that makes some American forensic dentists—the word *dentist* comes from Latin—just roll their eyes).

Rolling his eyes is one of the most dramatic expressions you'll ever see on the face of forensic odontologist Dr. Lowell Levine, who is as spare on gestures as he is with words. Dr. Levine keeps to himself with an extraordinary sense of cool. It is a trait I value, especially since we are co-directors at the New York State Police Medico-Legal Investigations Unit.

When the bite marks of Ted Bundy, the serial killer finally convicted and executed in Florida, brought dental impression evidence to the consciousness of America, Levine was right there. He testified for the prosecution in that case. Since then he has been involved in the identification of the Romanovs; the exhumation, identification and determination of the cause and manner of death of the "disappeared ones" in Argentina; the identification of Nazi war criminal Joseph Mengele; the trial of sportscaster Marv Albert; and the medico-legal investigations of many of the recent U.S. airline disasters, including TWA 800, which exploded and plunged into the waters off Long Island.

I have worked with Dr. Levine for more than thirty years, and while many images of him stay with me, the one that I immediately recall is at the Flight 800 investigation. Airline crashes are scenes of unfathomable chaos. Many people imagine that a plane crash is like a big funeral home, with dead bodies lying about. It's not. Airline crashes are ravaged and dispersed scenes of plane parts and bits of luggage, initially indistinguishable body parts, smoke and fire and charred evidence. They are cacophonous, swarming with police and emergency squads and people carrying all manner of law enforcement and investigative gear, badges, hats and vests—and right in the middle of it all you will find Lowell Levine and other forensic dentists, quietly doing their job.

In cases like that the forensic odontologist may be working with fragments of human remains in order to identify the dead. It is the same with the investigations our country makes all over the world to bring home whatever might be found of those lost in the wars we have fought. Amid the tiny fragments of tooth and bone may be found a bridge, a wedge of a gold crown, a piece of porcelain, a molar—anything from which an impression may be made and matched to answer the questions that come with unnatural death.

Other parts of the head tell other stories. Sometimes there are questions that can be answered only by analysis of the most slender forensic evidence the head provides: the human hair. Such was the case of the death investigation of Diana, Princess of Wales.

Inevitably people will theorize endlessly about the deaths of Diana, Dodi Al Fayed and their chauffeur, Henri Paul. Typing any combination of their names into an Internet search box reveals hundreds of links to conspiracy theories regarding what happened that night. But theorizing is unnecessary, for it is the plain and tragic fact that as Henri Paul was racing a luxury Mercedes-Benz through the streets of Paris on a hot summer night in 1997, a large amount of drugs and alcohol was coursing through his veins.

We know this from the history of Henri Paul's drug use that showed up like a timeline in his hair. After the crash, blood analysis quickly revealed that Henri Paul had a high level of alcohol in his body; his hair later revealed the alcohol rehabilitation drugs he had also been taking.

At autopsy, hairs were plucked from Henri Paul's head. They were tested by dissolving them in a solvent to release the drugs that were present. Hair analysis now permits us to identify many substances that get into the hair bulb from the bloodstream and then remain locked in the hair shaft as it grows. These include heroin, cocaine, nicotine, caffeine, Prozac, marijuana, digitalis and the newer date rape drugs.

Such science represents a recent advance in criminalistics. Not long ago, hair analysis was limited to visually comparing under the microscope hair found at a crime scene with hair from a particular individual. The examiner would consider a variety of factors, including color, coarseness, granule distribution, hair diameter and the presence or absence of a medulla. Many of these identifications turned out to be wrong when DNA analyses of the hairs were conducted.

Each hair on your body grows out of a tiny skin pocket called a follicle. The base of each hair is attached to the follicle by what is known as the root bulb. Each strand of hair has three layers: the medulla, which runs the length of the hair; the cortex, which contains the pigment granules, which, in turn, are important points of comparison among samples; and the cuticle, which is the hair's outer covering.

The simplest differences among hair may also be the most striking: African hair tends to be curly and contains unevenly distributed microscopic pigment granules; Caucasian hair is usually straight or wavy with more evenly distributed pigment granules; and among Asians, the medulla tends to be a long, continuous tube, unlike other races, which tend to have medullas that are fragmented. (In some non-Asians, the medulla may even be absent.) Animal hair, which provides warmth as well as color, is distinguished by a thicker medulla and cuticle than those of human origin.

The use of hair as a specimen to detect cocaine was first reported in 1981. Now that procedure is widespread. Hair testing for drugs offers distinct advantages over urine testing. Hair is easier to collect and store. It is externally available. And, it can provide information on the individual's history of drug use.

Each month, human head hair typically grows one centimeter (or almost half an inch). So a strand taken from the scalp can be read like a timeline. To determine when a drug was taken, the hair is cut into one-centimeter lengths, each of which is individually tested. Interestingly, considerable differences in trace element and drug concentrations have been reported in hair samples collected from different locations on the body. Morphine concentrations, for instance, have been found to be highest in pubic hair, followed by armpit or axillary hair, then scalp hair. Methadone concentrations have been found to be highest in armpit or axillary hair, followed by pubic hair and then scalp hair. Samples for cocaine testing are usually taken from the scalp, as are any samples where drug use over time is an issue. An adequate sample for testing is approximately one hundred milligrams of hair, cut as closely to the scalp as possible from a live person or plucked from the scalp of the dead. The root ends are then closely aligned so that the hair strands can be cut accurately for segmental analysis.

Laboratory workers will then wash the hair sample to remove lipids, oils, cosmetics and any adhering drug, and cut it into one-centimeter sections. The hair is then digested in a solution with an enzyme or base, depending on the drugs being sought. A screening test then uses antibodies that bind the drugs in the digested hair. If this preliminary test shows that drugs are present, a confirmation test is done, in which the drug is separated from other compounds by a method called chromatography. The hair is then placed in a mass spectrometer and vaporized into components, allowing small amounts of the drug and its breakdown products to be analyzed.

The hair on the head of Henri Paul revealed that for several months prior to his death, he had been taking "therapeutic" amounts of fluoxetine, the generic name for the antidepressant Prozac, as well as Tiapride. Both drugs are used in the treatment of chronic alcoholism.

Blood alcohol concentration (BAC) is the amount of alcohol in the bloodstream. It is measured in percentages. A reading of .10—the threshold of legal intoxication in many states—means that the drinker has one part alcohol per one thousand parts of blood. BAC can be measured in the breath, blood or urine, and while most people commonly associate this level with drunk driving, it would be a great public health leap forward if, instead, we set our standards lower. In many countries it has been lowered to .05. This lower limit could prevent many thousands of deaths and injuries each year in our country.

The drugs that we know Henri Paul consumed can enhance the detrimental effects of alcohol in impairing judgment, can blur vision and can slow reaction time—in short, can diminish one's ability to drive a car. And tragically, they did. Blood tests at autopsy revealed that at the time of death, Paul had a BAC between .175 and .187, which is nearly four times the French legal blood alcohol threshold of .05. This is the equivalent of the alcohol content of eight or nine shots of straight whiskey, eight or nine twelve-ounce cans of beer, or eight or nine four-ounce glasses of wine.

Toxicologic analysis of blood for its alcohol content is simple: If the person is alive, alcohol content metabolizes away at about one shot per hour. After death, the alcohol metabolism stops, and alcohol remains trapped in the blood at its level at the time of death.

It was not until September 1999—a little more than two years after the crash that took the three lives—that a Paris judge placed responsibility for the accident on Henri Paul. That ruling dismissed charges against nine photographers and one motorcycle courier who had pursued the car and who were originally blamed by many for the crash. The judge's report stated that although the pack had imposed a "continuous and insistent presence" on Dodi Al Fayed and Diana since the couple had arrived in Paris a few hours before the accident, "the driver of the car was inebriated and under the effect of drugs incompatible with alcohol. He was not in a position to maintain control of the vehicle."

Years after his death, Napoleon Bonaparte's hair and the analysis of his hair remain a subject of hot debate among conspiracy theorists and historians.

Napoleon Bonaparte died in 1821, at the age of fifty-one, following a lengthy illness. An autopsy was performed by his physicians, and a large cancer of the stomach was discovered and determined to be the cause of his death.

Despite this, some assassination buffs say he was poisoned in some subtle way by either his French attendants or his English captors. Samples of his hair were known to exist, and in 1962, they were tested. Arsenic was found, and a conspiracy theory emerged.

Among physicians, arsenic had long been known as "inheritance powder," because it was a favorite among family poisoners. It is highly toxic, colorless, odorless and found in household items such as pesticides and herbicides. The grayish white powder is also an ingredient in pigments and is contained in pressurized lumber (and will be released if the wood is burned).

A person can be accidentally poisoned by arsenic through inhalation, absorption through the skin or mucous membranes, skin contact and ingestion. People have died by breathing arsenic fumes, licking paintbrushes to make a fine point, or wearing inadequate clothing when applying arsenic-based products. The effects of mild poisoning from inhalation include loss of appetite, nausea and diarrhea. Effects of more severe chronic or acute exposure include skin lesions, chronic headaches, apathy, a garlic odor on the breath, a metallic taste in the mouth, a bronzing pigment of the skin resembling "raindrops on a dusty road" and possible damage to the liver. In addition, arsenic and arsenic compounds are known cancer-causing agents and have been implicated in lung and skin cancer and associated with birth defects.

But arsenic was not the cause of Napoleon's death. In fact, the arsenic in the emperor's hair was found in such small quantities that it might have come from the wallpaper in his bedroom or from the groundwater that he drank during his exile. The fact is, arsenic is in all of us, since it is one of the most abundant element in the earth's soil and is present in all living organisms. It is not harmful in these naturally occurring levels.

But many people in the nineteenth century were poisoned by vapors from the arsenic dyes in the green pigments of their wallpaper. The colors Scheele's green and Paris green are both derived from arsenic compounds and were widely used in paint and wallpaper after 1780. Not until 1893 was it discovered that the vapors produced by damp walls or moldy wallpaper released the volatile substance trimethylarsenic into the air.

Well-authenticated pieces of wallpaper from Napoleon's rooms during his exile reveal that its design of green rosettes contained about one-third of a gram of arsenic per square meter. This amount of arsenic probably did little more than affect Napoleon's aesthetic senses, but it was certainly enough to account for the traces found in his hair.

Of course, the beautiful wallpaper continued to be in vogue. In the late 1950s I was present when a call came into Bellevue Hospital regarding Clare Boothe Luce, then the newly appointed American ambassador to Rome. She had fallen ill in Rome and was in search of her New York physician, who was attending at the hospital where I was an intern. As it turned out, she had been inhaling the Paris green wallpaper fumes in her new residence in Rome. (Some of the newspapers suggested that her illness was a Russian plot, but it wasn't.)

Place your hands on either side of your head with the tips of your thumbs just inside your ears and the tips of your pinkies touching your lower eyelashes. Now picture an imaginary reference plane passing from the center of the ear hole through the bottom of the eyeball socket. This is known as the Frankfurt plane. When the head tilts forward, the Frankfurt plane tilts with it.

The Frankfurt plane is important in learning the identity of an unknown skull. When a facial reconstruction is needed, it will be the job of a forensic artist to get the angle just right; only then can he or she begin working with the skull. Theirs is intimate work done in a solitary office: an artist, working in three dimensions, trying to regenerate a human identity.

The artist will place the skull on a special work stand that allows the skull to be tilted until it is situated in the Frankfurt horizontal position, making the Frankfurt plane line up along the horizon.

Much of what makes us appear unique is the depth of our tissue over specific points on our skulls. These human facial tissue depth points have been studied and collected over the years using methods ranging from needle insertion into the dead (which eventually proved less than precise since the dead are lying down and tissue flattens) to the use of sonograms on the living. As a result, we know the normal depth on thirty-two sites on the human face and the variations by race, gender and age.

These sites are known as anchor points. The forensic artist will plot out those points on the skull using rubber erasers the approximate size of those found on a number two pencil, which are cut to the individual anchor point depths and glued directly to the bone. Each eraser will bear the number of the corresponding anchor point across its top.

Artificial eyes are then placed in the skull's sockets, centered at the proper depth. To discourage influencing a viewer in any way, neutral tones are chosen for the irises. Then clay will be systematically applied at the depths marked by the erasers, following the contours of the skull. Any knowledge of the lifestyle of the person is taken into account. Did he wear glasses, for instance? They may have affected the shape of the temple and the ears, as well as the bridge of the nose. Did he smoke a pipe? This will offset the jaw. Various measurements will be made to determine the thickness of the nose, and the length and thickness of the mouth. Even the geographic location of where the deceased lived and the details of his lifestyle—sun exposure literally tans the skin, smoking caves in the sinuses and missing teeth sink the cheeks—all show up on the face and will be factored into its reconstruction.

Aging causes changes to the face that may be unattractive and are governed by gravity: Ears and chins lengthen, but dimples always remain in place. The mouth sinks. Flesh hangs. It's human nature.

What amazes me is how much human physiology is known to the people who do facial reconstruction. They are not doctors, after all. They are artists. And yet they know more than most physicians about the workings of the face and head.

For instance, the subtle differences of each muscle are known to professional facial reconstructionists and precisely guide their work. This requires exacting skill, since the muscles of the human face and cranium are divided into groups based on their positions on the head: the cranial region, auricular region, palpebral region, orbital region, nasal region, maxillary region, mandibular region and intermaxillary region. Within these groups the muscles are layered together according to the tasks they perform—whether it be squinting, chewing, screaming or any of the other things the face and head can do. Facial muscles also serve the higher function of expressing emotion.

Wigs fill in for hair. Glasses will be supplied, and after much work, there will again be a face over the skull.

It is an exacting, meticulous science, sometimes too much so: Loved ones frequently take one look and say, "Nope, not him," all too quickly. (On the contrary, when families are brought down to see a family member in the morgue, they are *all* too ready to say, "It's him," when sometimes it isn't. Once they have been told by the police that someone is dead, they believe it and sometimes cover their eyes and confirm the identification without ever looking at the body.)

"Two-dimensional reconstructions" are actually sketches. While they hold less allure for the moviegoers, they are the preferred method for many forensic artists. Sketches seem to make people look and react in a less literal way: "Well, it kind of looks like the guy down the street," they might say. "And it also looks like so-and-so." And all of a sudden there are two leads where there were none.

A two-dimensional reconstruction starts with an unidentified skull, then uses the same data and tissue markers. But then the skull is photographed at its profile and frontal views. The photos are enlarged to life size and then taped, always in the Frankfurt horizontal position, next to one another. A transparent vellum sheet is placed over each. Then the sketching begins with the artist using the tissue markers as contour indicators, and also using any geographical and lifestyle information.

Checking the website of any county medical examiner's office may reveal the finished product of such work. The Hamilton County medical examiner in Chattanooga, Tennessee, for instance, recently ran as many as twelve versions of the same reconstructed face of an adult white female—dark hair, light hair, short hair, long hair, glasses on, glasses off, hair up, hair down, straight hair, wavy hair—in an effort to get someone to identify a body found along the southbound side of Interstate 24.

The photographs were accompanied by a profile—age, race, sex, height, weight, and description, as well as the category of "other": the presence of a red, "twist-style" ponytail holder and a rubber band around the left wrist and the possibility of a "peculiar stride" in life, owing to possible bowleggedness or a limp due to an old lower extremity fracture, for which old X rays would be the identifier.

The site also included a list of what is called "antemortem traumas"—injuries that occurred before death—including a healed fracture of the left cuboid, which would result from an injury to the top of the left foot, possibly causing the limp. Other antemortem traumas included injuries to the right foot and the outside of the left hand, a healed fracture to the right first rib and healed fractures of the nose. From this evidence, it is reasonable to conclude someone had been beating this woman for years.

The images ran in the *Chattanooga Times Free Press,* complete with the web address, adding yet another tool to the investigation—the Internet. Thus the techniques involved in bringing that one woman's identity back to her and her remains back to her family spanned generations of knowledge, from anatomy to dental impression analysis to hair analysis, all the way to the Internet.

In the last few years, positive matches have been made from other parts of the human head, and as a result, new methods are being added to the already varied toolbox of the criminalist. In England, for instance, the police have been compiling the world's largest computer database of ear prints, with plans to use them in the same way as fingerprint evidence in linking suspects to crimes.

It has been a long time coming. In the latter half of the 1700s, Johann Caspar Lavater (1741–1801) studied and recorded the individualized designs of the ear. One hundred years later, fingerprints were developed and were enjoying wide use by criminalists. At that time they were supplemented by the use of photography to record physical images of criminals. Standard procedure in Europe was the Bertillon system, which required measuring specific parts of the body. Although that eventually fell out of favor, a lot had been noted and learned about the identifiable differences among humans, and to some, the ear remained of particular interest.

It was an American named Alfred Iannarelli who designed what some consider the standard work on ear prints, including a classification system. A former deputy sheriff in Alameda County, California, Iannarelli first got interested in the ear in the 1940s and later published two editions of a book on "earology," or the science of ear identification.

To date, ear prints as well as lip prints—which are also unique to each individual—have not been accepted in America's courts because they have not been generally accepted in the scientific community. But while no one expects them to replace fingerprints, they are still collected when found and have been used to place individuals at crime scenes.

Although the newer sciences always add something to the palette of the criminalist, they rarely remove anything. Science doesn't replace science in the pursuit of justice; it adds to the existing body of knowledge. The sciences weave together and help us in our work: The knowledge of the formation of the bones and overlying muscles of the head helps an artist produce an image that may look like someone whose hair samples, X rays or bite mark impressions may be on record and may be matched after a facial image is put on a website by the police.

The ability to synthesize this information is the job of the forensic scientist—and good ones do it well. This only confirms for me that amid the wonders of the human head, it is the human mind that is the most astonishing wonder of all.

Ten

JUNK

Fred Zain was a forensic science superstar. By all accounts he was amazing—astonishing, it seemed—in his ability to find things that no one else could find: infinitesimal flecks of blood overlooked by everyone else, tiny blots of semen unnoticed by every other examiner. Not only were his eyes good, but his lab results time and again produced genetic markers in the kind of indictable numbers that district attorneys only dare to dream about. As a result, he was sought after by prosecutors who wanted to get convictions in difficult cases. He was driven; he was successful. He wanted to win in the worst way.

Which is exactly what he did.

Between 1977 and 1993, Fred Zain tested and testified about blood and semen evidence in hundreds of murder and rape trials. His work primarily involved cases in Texas and West Virginia, but the referrals he accepted later in his career brought him to Hawaii,

Delaware, Kentucky, Nebraska, New Mexico, Ohio, Pennsylvania and Virginia.

He began his expert witness career in West Virginia, where he worked in the serology division of the state police crime lab from 1977 until 1989, in the later years as head of serology. He rapidly rose through the state police ranks from trooper to corporal, sergeant and lieutenant. His stature led to a job offer in another state, and he moved away, leaving behind an astonishing record of convictions.

One of those convicted was Glen Woodall, who in 1987 was found guilty of first-degree sexual assault, first-degree sexual abuse, kidnapping and aggravated robbery of two women.

In separate incidents, the two women had been abducted at knifepoint in a shopping mall parking lot. Both times the assailant wore a ski mask and forced his victims to close their eyes during the attack. In the first attack, the man drove around in the woman's car, repeatedly raped her and stole a gold watch and five dollars. Against his wishes, she briefly opened her eyes and noted that her assailant wore brown pants and that he was uncircumcised. The details of the second attack, as well as what the victim noticed, were nearly the same.

During the pretrial hearing, the judge denied a defense request for an "experimental new" DNA test of the defendant's blood and semen samples and those from the victims' clothing. The denial was based on the defense's inability to offer any expert testimony on the new test's validity or reliability.

At Woodall's trial, Fred Zain testified that based upon his scientific analysis of the semen recovered from the victims, the assailant's blood type was identical to Woodall's. The jury was convinced. Woodall was sentenced to two life terms without parole and to 203 to 335 years in prison, to be served consecutively.

After the trial, the defense raised the DNA issue again. A DNA test was performed, but the court held that the results were inconclusive. On July 6, 1989, the West Virginia Supreme Court of Appeals affirmed the conviction.

But eventually, after several appeal petitions, the state supreme court allowed the evidence in the Woodall case to be released for additional DNA testing. Zain, by then, had been promoted and had moved on, but DNA had also moved on to a higher rank in criminal investigation.

The testing done in the subsequent habeas corpus proceeding established that Woodall could not have been the assailant. His conviction was overturned. In 1992, after serving five years for crimes he did not commit, Woodall was freed. He sued the state of West Virginia for wrongful imprisonment and false conviction and received one million dollars in settlement. The reversal of his conviction sparked an investigation into the science done in the lab by Fred Zain.

Four hundred years ago, Sir Francis Bacon entitled his seminal work on the subject of science *Novum Organum*. Loosely translated from the Latin, it means "a new instrument," in this case, a new instrument of reasoning. Bacon wrote: "The human understanding is not a dry light, but is infused by desire and emotion, which give rise to 'wishful science.' For man prefers to believe what he wants to be true. He therefore rejects difficulties, being impatient of inquiry; sober things, because they restrict his hope; deeper parts of nature, because of his superstition; the light of experience, because of his arrogance and pride, lest his mind should seem to concern itself with things mean and transitory; things that are strange and contrary to all expectation, because of common opinion. In short, emotion in numerous, often imperceptible ways pervades and infects the understanding."

Others have furthered our understanding of the impact of

"wishful science" on the pursuit of pure knowledge. Nobel Prize–winning chemist Irving Langmuir coined the term *pathological science,* for "the science of things that aren't so," and Richard Feynman, a Nobel winner for his work in physics, focused on the source of the trouble when he warned, "The first principle is that you must not fool yourself and you're the easiest person to fool."

Perhaps scientists initially fool themselves all the time, as Albert Einstein is often quoted, "If we knew what we were doing, it would not be called research, would it?" But good scientists don't fool themselves for long and never go on to fool others: Long before they speak about what they think they see, they retest, reevaluate and review their results from every angle. And then they speak or publish—or, in my case, go to court—each time hoping to further the truth.

I agree with Linus Pauling, who once said, "Science is the search for the truth—it is not a game in which one tries to best his opponent, to do harm to others." Science is a tool, and despite the fact that it has been used to do so, science is not a blunt object meant to be wielded by one set of interests against another. It is not to be taken lightly, manipulated or misrepresented. Whether it be the false hope of patients in a new cure, the misplaced funding and awarding of prizes for scientific research or the wrongful conviction of the innocent, the consequences of bad science can be dire.

Much as I hate to admit it, the sad fact is that some forensic scientists do, indeed, fool a lot of the people a lot of the time.

What motivations lead them to do so may be as individual as the people involved: greed, stress, naïveté, ambition, fear, money—who can say? In my line of work, it may be that there is an overzealous prosecutor breathing down your neck for some conclusive indictable evidence. Maybe you've got tickets to the opera or to a vacation in France and you simply can't put in the time to check your results. Maybe your wife is in a difficult pregnancy or your husband has committed tax fraud. Maybe you just like to win, or you don't really know your science as well as you think you do.

In my line of work, I think most sloppy scientists are simply trying to please their employers—whichever side they are working with. They feel as if they are part of a team—prosecution or defense—and they want to be a team player when, in fact, their obligation as a scientist should preclude that. By becoming part of a team they become advocates for that side.

Whatever the motivation, when bad forensic science is done, justice is going to suffer: Someone is going to get away with something (murder, perhaps), or the wrong person is going to pay for another's crime.

There is work that is done well and work which, done by the wrong set of hands before the wrong pair of eyes, simply turns the science into junk. Bad science can happen in even the best of the solid sciences because none of the disciplines is immune to the ego, habits, practices, needs, desires, ambition, zeal or just plain stupidity of someone who practices bad science.

Junk happens.

The Union of Concerned Scientists in Cambridge, Massachusetts, which may have coined the phrase, defines junk science as "work presented as valid science that falls outside the rigors of the scientific method and the peer review process."

I would also include dressing up speculation in scientific terms to make things that are not proven sound as though they are. When people do that, they are giving the appearance of science when the work isn't scientific. To me, junk science is wishful thinking wrapped in a pseudoscientific cloak; in my world, I see everything from bad science to questionable science.

Junk science is not new. Much of today's junk may have been yesterday's accepted truths. Consider the case of phrenology, for instance. In its heyday it was considered a solid science, the identification of basic brain functions as determined by cranial features. The shape and features of the head and face determined aspects of behavior. In the 1840s there were international conferences of phrenologists as well as professional associations. Today we know this to be quackery.

An effort to keep out junk was one of the forces behind the U.S. Supreme Court's *Daubert* ruling of 1993. With *Daubert,* the Court intended to tighten the standards applied to determining the quality of expert testimony by an expert witness. The ruling was meant to weed out unqualified expert testimony because it changed the admissibility of testimony in at least two significant ways: First, by basing the test for admissibility of evidence on "scientific knowledge"—not merely general acceptance in a particular field, but whether proof of "reliability" of a technique or scientific method could be established; and second, by giving the determination of reliability to the trial judges.

In spite of *Daubert,* I see, hear and read about junk, bad and pathological forensic science all the time. I come up against it in court when an "expert" desires to stretch the limits of what a specific science can tell us or when the so-called expert has little or no expertise on the topic at hand but tries to testify to it anyway. *Daubert* has not stopped junk, bad and pathological science from helping to send innocent people to prison. In the most tragic circumstances of all, I see junk science wielded in capital punishment cases, sometimes putting people who my science tells me are innocent on death row. There can be no worse feeling than watching an innocent person be found guilty—let alone sentenced to death.

Despite *Daubert,* junk science is still getting its day in court because while we have tried to regulate what comes before a judge and jury, we have neglected to professionalize the credentials of those who do the science.

For example, the Centers for Disease Control (CDC) estimate that medical examiners or coroners investigate 20 percent of the approximately two million deaths which occur in America each year. Investigation practices vary among jurisdictions but generally break down to 22 states currently using the medical examiner system, 11 using coroners and 17 using a combination of both. In the state of New York, for instance, there are 62 counties, of which about 50 employ coroners and 12 employ medical examiners.

Half of America's counties employ medical examiners, all of whom are physicians. But fewer than four hundred are trained forensic pathologists. The other half of the counties employ coroners, most of whom are untrained in medicine. Frequently they are undertakers. Some are plumbers, bookkeepers and, only occasionally, doctors. Is it any wonder, then, that good science is often absent from America's courts?

After establishing a winning record in West Virginia, Fred Zain, the former forensic science superstar, got a job offer to become the chief of physical evidence in Bexar County, Texas. He moved to San Antonio in 1989.

That same year Jack Davis was arrested for the sexual assault, murder and mutilation of Kathie Balonis, of New Braunfels, Texas, a community just north of San Antonio. At the time of the murder, Davis was employed as a maintenance man at Balonis's apartment complex. There were no witnesses to the crime.

Zain testified at Davis's trial that blood specimens found under the body of the victim came from Davis. Davis was convicted of murder, and the Texas jury came within one vote of sentencing him to death. In 1992, a hearing was convened to investigate prosecutorial misconduct in the Davis case. In a deposition, again under oath, Zain changed his testimony and stated that the blood samples in question actually belonged to the victim. By that time Davis had served four years of his life sentence in prison. He was freed.

Back in West Virginia, the state supreme court had, by this time, ordered an investigation into the entire body of work by its former state police serologist. The result of that investigation was an unprecedented published opinion by the court concluding that the actual guilt of 134 people was substantively in doubt because the convictions were based on the work of Fred Zain.

One of the reasons the court's investigation had to be so thorough is that bad science contaminates everything around it.

It certainly did in the case of William Harris. As a talented state champion athlete and student, Harris was a teenager whose peers respected him both on and off the field. He was a high school senior with the promise of college scholarships and a bright future ahead of him. And then, in 1985, his life tragically intersected with the bad science of Fred Zain.

A woman living near Harris was sexually assaulted by a person she described as young, male, athletic and black. Other than those broad characteristics, Harris did not fit the other details of her description. And, according to the original police report, the victim eliminated him in a photo lineup, stating that she knew Harris was not her attacker.

The police report on the photo lineup in which the victim excluded Harris never surfaced at his trial. (In fact it only came to light in a civil suit more than a decade later.) Zain's faulty scientific evidence linked Harris to the crime. And it is possible that when the faulty evidence was shared with investigating deputies as well as with the victim, it reinforced the police's belief that her original elimination of Harris must have been wrong.

The victim may have been influenced by the faulty evidence, as well, because at trial, she unhesitatingly identified Harris as her assailant, testifying that there was "no doubt" in her mind. Her testimony was supported by that of a deputy sheriff, who testified about the subsequent live lineup, stating for the record that not only had the victim picked Harris out, but that she had started to cry when she saw Harris and that she had then said, "There was no question, that was absolutely him."

Harris was convicted and sentenced to a ten-to-twenty-year term in the maximum security West Virginia penitentiary. He was released in 1995, after seven years in prison, when DNA testing confirmed his innocence.

No convictions are based solely on science, and none of Fred Zain's convictions were made only on his findings. But some of Zain's convictions were obtained after nonscientific evidence of guilt was bolstered or exaggerated following exposure of the witness to the fraudulent scientific evidence.

Bad science therefore can contaminate more than scientific evidence when it influences others. My experience has shown me that even when the erroneous scientific evidence is exposed, the prosecution will be disinclined to retreat, often believing that the error was harmless because of the nonscientific evidence also available.

What traditionally happens in these cases is that no effort is made by the criminal justice system to identify how the mistakes that resulted in a false conviction were made or how they can be prevented in the future. As often happens when a false conviction is discovered, police and prosecutors as well as the victim's family continue to believe they had the right person but that he was let off on a technicality. There will be no search for the real perpetrator.

The West Virginia Supreme Court stated in its report on Zain's misconduct that his behavior included "overstating the strength of results; . . . reporting inconclusive results as conclusive; . . . repeatedly altering laboratory records." The report also noted that Zain's irregularities were "the result of systematic practice rather than occasional inadvertent error," and stated that his "supervisors may have ignored or concealed complaints of his misconduct." However, no one else was punished.

Although cases of laboratory fraud are not unique to the state of West Virginia—recently there have been public charges that Joyce Gilchrist, an Oklahoma City police chemist, gave erroneous testimony (which she denies) for many years, including in many death penalty cases—the Zain case appears to be the first time that an American appellate court has discredited a forensic scientist's entire career and authorized the reopening, in habeas corpus proceedings, of every case he has handled.

Many convicted persons were permitted to file a writ of habeas corpus to review evidence if Zain worked on their cases. Gerald Wayne Davis is one convicted man who did just that.

In May 1986, Davis was convicted by a jury in Kanawha County, West Virginia, of kidnapping and sexual assault. The circuit court judge sentenced him to fourteen to thirty-five years in prison. Also convicted in the case was his father, Dewey Davis, who was found guilty of abduction, first-degree sexual abuse and second-degree sexual assault.

The victim had testified that on February 18, 1986, she had dropped off her laundry at the Davis home and that when she returned to pick it up, she was attacked and raped by the younger Davis on his water bed. She further claimed that his father was present during the attack and made no efforts to intervene on her behalf.

Among the evidence was testimony by a state police chemist that DNA tests could not exclude Davis as the source of the semen found on the victim's clothing.

Following the Zain investigation, the Davis writ was granted to perform DNA testing on the remaining trial evidence. Those tests showed that the DNA on the clothing was definitely not from Davis. A second series of tests was run. They, too, excluded Davis. As a result the convictions were annulled. The charges against his father were dismissed, but the prosecution wanted to retry Gerald Davis. Finally, on December 4, 1995, a Kanawha County Circuit Court jury deliberated for just ninety minutes before acquitting Davis. By that time each man had served eight years in prison.

In 1993 Fred Zain was dismissed from his job in San Antonio after evidence in a murder case was lost, and Bexar County Medical Examiner Vincent DiMaio ordered an extensive review of Zain's San Antonio work.

The estimates of the number of cases that Fred Zain worked on in his career range from 1,500 to 4,500. In its report on what might be the most egregious case of forensic science fraud in American history, the West Virginia Supreme Court of Appeals concluded that "as a matter of law, any testimonial or documentary evidence offered by Zain at any time in any criminal prosecution should be deemed invalid, unreliable, and inadmissible in determining whether to award a new trial in any habeas corpus proceeding."

The timing of Fred Zain's move to the Lone Star State and his subsequent work there overlaps the years of practice of another forensic scientist in Texas whose findings will also cause repercussions for years to come. In fact, estimates are that it could easily be the year 2020 before the appeals and writs citing the work of Dr. Ralph Erdmann cease to flow through court.

Ralph Erdmann was a forensic pathologist who performed as many as four hundred autopsies in capital as well as noncapital cases each year during the 1980s in Texas. While it may never be fully known just how much bad science he practiced, gruesome details of his tenure emerged after one family read the autopsy report of a loved one, in which Erdmann stated that the deceased's spleen had been removed and examined and weighed as part of the procedure. They doubted it: The deceased person's spleen had been removed years before. As a result, the family intervened, and the body was exhumed. And when examined, the body was intact. No autopsy had been done, even though Erdmann had filed and testified to a full autopsy report.

At that point, a special prosecutor was appointed to look into Erdmann's work. What emerged were stories of faked autopsies and a report of a misplaced head and parts from two different bodies showing up in the same container. Among the most tragic of his mistakes, however, was the case of Terri Trosper, who had died in 1991.

Ralph Erdmann initially concluded that Trosper had choked on her own vomit. Her family didn't think so and sued, contending that he had botched her autopsy. When her body was exhumed, a second coroner determined that the mother of four daughters had, in fact, been smothered in a vicious assault. In April 1992, a Texas jury sentenced her former lover Ricky Bradford to life in prison for her murder.

A ruling in the family's suit ordered Erdmann to pay a $250,000 default payment to Trosper's family. When notification of the suit was sent to Erdmann in Kirkland, Washington, where he had moved, he failed to respond, forcing the judge to make the default ruling in the Trosper case. At the time, Erdmann actually was serving three concurrent sentences in a Lubbock jail for botching seven autopsies in northwest Texas. Trosper's autopsy was not one of the seven. A recent count totaled ten civil suits similar to Trosper's in Lubbock County alone. In his career Erdmann was responsible for death investigations in forty-eight counties in the state of Texas.

At one of his court hearings, Erdmann testified that "I'm human and can do errors, yes. But intentionally? Never."

Who was he fooling? Himself, as Richard Feynman warned us? The public? All people concerned, all of the time?

In 1994 he pleaded no contest to seven felonies tied to falsified evidence and botched autopsies in three counties. He surrendered his medical license and was sentenced to ten years' probation, two hundred hours of community service and repayment of $17,000 in autopsy fees. He moved to Washington State, where police later reportedly found a cache of more than a hundred guns in his home, including an illegally owned M-16 assault rifle. It was that conviction that caused the revocation of the Texas probations. He served two years in prison, after which he was released and moved to San Antonio.

But the damage done by Ralph Erdmann's bad science was not over. In 1998, a father whose fourteen-month-old child had died nine years before had his worst suspicions confirmed. The exhumation and a second autopsy of his son's body revealed that the child had not died of pneumonia, as stated on the death certificate, but that the boy had been murdered.

For nine years the friends and family of Norman Ballard had urged him to get on with his life, to put his son's death aside and move on. But Ballard had nagging suspicions that he couldn't shake. And then, in 1998, new witnesses went to the police with tips that the baby may have been slain. The case was turned over to a Texas Ranger, who was initially skeptical—until he saw the signature at the bottom of the autopsy report: Ralph Erdmann.

As the stories poured out, it was revealed that Erdmann was sloppy, messy and disorganized on his best days, and that he routinely said he had performed autopsies that, in fact, he hadn't. To some, it sounded like ineptitude. But it is the nature of the scientist's work that he must document his findings in the form of autopsy reports. Erdmann repeatedly falsified them in order to support prosecution arguments. And he did so in some cases that resulted in the death penalty. That is not mere ineptitude. That is pathological science.

After the investigation into Erdmann's work, the special prosecutor concluded, "If the prosecution theory was that death was caused by a Martian death ray, then that was what Dr. Erdmann reported."

He was fooling everyone, it seemed, until someone finally raised the issue of his expertise.

To fully understand the impact of the science practiced by Erdmann and Zain, you must look at each case within its geographical context. Both of these men, remember, committed some of their worst science in Texas.

Texas was one of the first states to rewrite and reenact its death penalty law after the United Sates Supreme Court ruled capital punishment constitutional in 1972. The following year the Texas legislature passed a new capital murder statute that required juries to answer certain questions during the punishment phase. When the law reinstating the death penalty was passed in 1976, it included the provision that Texas jurors be required to determine whether there is a probability that the defendant "would commit criminal acts of violence that would constitute a continuing threat to society." In fact, Texas is the only state in America that asks jurors a punishment question regarding whether a convict is likely to be a future danger to society. Death penalty opponents as well as some psychiatric experts say that predicting future dangerousness is junk science. Death penalty supporters say that determining the potential future violence of a convict is an essential element that has allowed juries some discretion in assessing death sentences—a decision the U.S. Supreme Court has said that juries may be able to make.

To determine future violence, the prosecutor in the case may call on an expert to speak to future mental health and possible behavior of those convicted. For many years in Texas, a prosecution favorite was Dr. James Grigson, a Dallas forensic psychiatrist, whose testimony in 124 capital cases contributed to 115 death sentences. That record earned him the nickname of "Dr. Death," used by both sides of the capital punishment issue.

After the guilt phase of his 1977 trial, Randall Dale Adams listened as Grigson referred to him as having a "sociopathic personality disorder," adding, "There is no question in my mind that Adams is guilty." During questioning as to whether Adams was likely to kill again in the future, given the opportunity, Grigson confidently offered his expert opinion: "He will kill again."

Film lovers may remember Randall Dale Adams as the subject of the documentary *The Thin Blue Line*. His wrongful conviction brought him within seventy-two hours of death in Texas. He was innocent and had never killed anyone.

Death penalty opponents say that though he lost twelve years of his life, he was lucky because he was one of the few wrongly accused who avoided execution. Death penalty supporters say that the system worked: He didn't die.

Is predicting the future behavior of the convicted junk science? Or is it bad science that has been institutionalized, reinforced, professionalized and now credentialed to justify the continuance of the death penalty? After all, as long as we continue to execute people, there will be a need to justify doing so by the findings of experts. And the expertise of those experts can be easily determined by looking at their credentials. Or can it?

There are forensic odontologists, handwriting experts, forensic geologists, botanists, document experts, forensic nurses, forensic accountants, forensic engineers, forensic psychiatrists, social workers, recorded evidence experts, the spectrum of psychological experts (including such subspecialties as subliminal message experts), wood experts, pollen experts, lip print experts and ear print experts among those who may be prepared to testify to something in court.

After *Daubert,* judges nationwide began to dismiss witnesses without proper credentials. "Experts," for their part, reacted by clamoring for places from which to get credentials. This, in turn, resulted in new credentialing organizations to help the court decide who is an expert by creating a voluntary peer review process known as board certification.

Unfortunately, there is no uniform set of standards in the forensic sciences for what constitutes the proper qualifications for such certification. Each specialty or subspeciality can create its own standards. As a result, there are widely ranging sets of credentials and credentialing offices. There are organizations such as the American Board of Document Examiners, for example, which requires that a candidate must have a bachelor's degree and at least two years' experience in a recognized lab and must also pass a three-part test: one part written, one part practical problem solving and one part oral. And experts must stand for recertification every five years.

There are also the "checkbook credentials," which, as the name implies, are simple—too simple—to get.

When Robert O'Block started out in the credentialing business in 1992, he was managing a handful of handwriting experts from a computer and two tables in his home in Branson, Missouri. He called his group the American Board of Handwriting Analysts and soon blitzed the forensic science world with glossy brochures, trying to recruit scientists to get their credentials from him. He soon renamed the group the American Board of Forensic Examiners, adorned his Jeep Cherokee with plates that read ABFE-1 and by 1994, paid himself $51,493. He installed a toll-free line (1-800-4A-Expert) for lawyers to call. In 1995, he again renamed the group, this time becoming the American College of Forensic Examiners.

At the outset, the credentialing process included a fee of $350 accompanying an application with résumés, professional licenses and details of experience, professional degrees and published articles. To receive their credentials, applicants had to achieve a score of at least 75 percent on a self-administered ethics test. The test could be taken up to three times, but it was waived for those with considerable experience.

Any candidate for board certification could also qualify for a waiver of the test by accumulating a certain number of points on the application. These points were self-awarded based on education, experience, knowledge, skills and training: 50 points for every doctorate held, 30 points for each master's degree and 20 for every bachelor's degree. Five points could be claimed for every year of experience, 10 for each article written and 5 for every scientific meeting attended in the previous ten years. It took as few as 100 points in some specialties to qualify for the waiver.

For those taking the ethics test, questions over the years have included:

In giving testimony at a deposition, it is appropriate to engage in shouting matches or arguments with abusive attorneys.

True or False?

In making your fee arrangement with a client, it is ethical to reduce your fee by 25 percent if your client does not obtain a favorable verdict in his favor at trial.

True or False?

If you're selling some of your forensic equipment and know about a subtle but serious problem in one piece, would you tell your prospective buyers?

Yes or No?

In 1997, O'Block's federal tax return listed his salary at $190,000. By the turn of the century, the American College of Forensic Examiners had a website, held an annual conference, boasted fifteen thousand members and totaled $2.2 million in annual revenue. It has become one of the largest credentialing bodies in forensic science. But the ACFE is only one of many such organizations, as can be seen by the ads littering the back pages of legal magazines.

Technology broadens the question of junk. For instance, forensic animation software has been around for a decade. It depends on the input of calculations of the factors involved—the bodies in motion in a car accident, for instance—to produce a reconstruction that can then be viewed and assessed by a jury. In the right hands, the software is a powerful scientific tool. But if erroneous assumptions are entered, the computer will generate images that are flawed. That is, as computer mavens have reminded us for a generation, "Junk in, junk out."

Software has the ability to provide a feeling for what *probably* happened at the crime scene by filling in sketchy evidence to yield an explanation. Is that misleading a jury or leading it effectively to a fair conclusion? After all, it depicts something we could only previously imagine. And once you picture something, it looks like the only possible version of events. But if there is a question about the personal ethics or devotion to scientific principles of those inputting the information, the possibility for manipulation is at least equal to that of any other forensic evidence.

Technology is a given in our lives. No one proposes that we do without it. But how do we live with it in the courtroom when many times a human life is in the hands of a jury whose minds are being influenced by what they are shown?

What juries can be shown is changing as fast as technology and judges allow, and as a result, juries will quickly come to expect moving, computerized crime scenes much as they now expect to see DNA evidence. In fact, the computerized moving images were used in the most recent of the Dr. Sam Sheppard trials in Cleveland in the year 2000.

The late Dr. Sheppard was found guilty in 1954 of murdering his wife, Marilyn. In a second trial he was found not guilty. This was the case that inspired the long-running television show *The Fugitive,* and every time an issue involving the Sheppards is back in the court, it shows up on television sets across America. It's one of those cases that goes on and on. In 2000, Sam, Dr. Sheppard's son, had a suit come to trial in what proved to be a futile attempt to have his father pronounced innocent—not just not guilty.

In that trial, lawyers for the opposing side used crime scene re-creation software to let the jurors tour the house via 3-D images shown on video monitors. Supporters of this technology argued that even though the video was based on old crime scene police photos—that its use provided a time machine of sorts—it allowed the jurors to feel as though they were moving about the place during the murder. After all, they could no longer take a tour of the scene of the crime; the real house had been demolished in the 1990s.

Just how often the wrong person is arrested is nothing short of astonishing. In a 1996 Justice Department report entitled "Convicted by Juries, Exonerated by Science: Case Studies in the Use of DNA Evidence to Establish Innocence After Trial," it was reported that in 8,048 rape and rape-and-murder cases referred to the FBI crime lab from 1988 until mid-1995, 2,012 of the primary suspects were exonerated by DNA evidence alone. Without that DNA testing, which was unavailable only a decade earlier, a significant number of those 2,012 would probably have been tried and convicted and would be serving time for crimes they did not commit.

DNA will go a long way toward preventing miscarriages of justice in the future since most wrongly suspected and accused people will be excluded during the initial testing of physical evidence, long before prosecution is even considered. DNA laboratory quality assurance and quality control protocols preclude the wholesale falsification of test results. And the miniscule amount of DNA material required for testing will ensure that there is enough to go around for outside labs to be used by the defense.

But there are no national standards of quality assurance for legal counsel. In fact, a recent national survey that looked at all capital murder sentences overturned since 1973 found that nearly 40 percent were reversed due to egregious incompetence on the part of the defense attorneys. Interestingly, a *Chicago Tribune* investigation published in 1999 found that since 1963, at least 381 homicide convictions nationwide have been overturned because overzealous prosecutors concealed evidence of innocence or presented evidence they knew to be false. Not one of those prosecutors has been convicted of any crime related to those convictions or barred from practicing law.

Most people convicted of capital offenses in this country are poor and are in no position to assemble "Dream Team" attorneys and hire expert witnesses to sift through the available crime science. The poor get public defenders who sometimes are handling a hundred cases at one time. We have set up a system where the surest safeguard against fraud and bias in criminal prosecutions is the threat of a good public defender. And while many of them are well meaning, determined, energetic and devoted public servants, they are also woefully underpaid and nearly always overworked. The public defender cannot be the defendant's only hope for good science when so many other professionals interact with the case along the way. And yet, in light of the lack of national professional standards, much of the burden for discovery of fraud, bias, bad science, junk, exaggeration and error falls onto the shoulders of those who are already under a huge burden: the public defenders who may be responsible for the initial defense as well as the appeal.

It was George Castelle, the chief public defender in Charleston, West Virginia, who represented the interests of all West Virginia prisoners in the 1993 special investigation of both Fred Zain and the West Virginia state police crime laboratory, nine of whose convictions have been overturned in whole or part, to date. Six have been freed. Castelle received a 1997 Reginald Heber Smith Award from the National Legal Aid and Defender Association for his role in exposing crime lab fraud and freeing those unjustly convicted through falsified scientific data. So the public defender system can work, burdened though it may be.

In Texas, however, elected judges appoint private attorneys to take on such cases. It is a system that is easily abused since some judges may be inclined to appoint friends, campaign contributors or those with a reputation for moving their cases swiftly along.

And yet Texas executes more people than any other state in America, forty alone in the year 2000. How many of those killed were, in fact, innocent? How many innocent people now sit on death row? Further, the fact is that less than 5 percent of murder cases involve DNA evidence, and nobody is focusing attention on the wrongfully convicted in cases where there is no DNA evidence. And while we read more every day about the wrongly accused awaiting execution, the question arises as to how many wrongly convicted people sit in jail for lesser crimes, convicted perhaps, on charges of robbery, burglary or aggravated assault. The stories of these people rarely make headlines. We may never know.

Eleven

RENO

If Wayne Newton is the star at the center of his own universe—and he is—then the jewels he wears are the planets that orbit in his pull: An eternity band, Saturn-like, bursting into rings of diamonds, adorns his wedding finger; a pinky ring soars in a mesmerizing constellation of color over his head as he croons; and a wristwatch is its own galaxy of platinum and precious stones.

As Wayne sings, his audience sees the trademark gestures of his long, tan hands in the light of the silvery sparkles of his accessories. But even the illusion of the heavens themselves does nothing to eclipse his stardom.

Type "Wayne Newton" into an Internet search box and you'll find more than forty thousand sites from which to choose (including www.waynenewton.com), many of which list his occupation as "singer." They're wrong. He is an entertainer; his voice is only part of the act. And they love him here in Reno, or more accurately, in Sparks, the city on the outskirts of Reno, smack up against the railroad yards in the darkened Celebrity Showroom of John Ascuaga's Nugget, the town's massive hotel and casino. He is singing to a packed house of people who, in their day jobs, are witnesses for the dead.

If scientists are skeptics, forensic scientists may be the mystics, because they can conjure up one human doing absolutely anything to his or her fellow man. After all, they have seen or heard of everything in the spectrum of human behavior. Once a year they meet, about 2,400 strong, to up the ante on our understanding of how badly we can behave: a new high-tech ligature; internet hits in the billions on kiddy porn; the first documented suicide by pneumatic hammer. They show one another their crime scene slides, comparing notes and talking about what's new in the world of unnatural death.

But right now it's the middle of their convention week, Wednesday afternoon, and they are listening to Wayne. And they love him.

He's scheduled to sing for forty-five minutes. But he plays for an hour and a half, during which time he snatches up or slides into a guitar, a banjo and a keyboard, extracting melody, rhythm and song from them with a showman's skill. He tells jokes, boogies, bends, drops to his knees and, yes, finally sings, "Danke Schoen," in the end converting even the mere voyeurs into fans. He seems to want the world to love him, to sing with him and laugh at his jokes ("I searched my brain deciding what to sing to this group— 'Dem Bones'? 'I'll Be Glad When You're Dead, You Rascal You'?" Laughter. "This is not a career move on my part, but when the world finds out I did this show they're going to say, 'I told you he was dead.'"). He thanks the crowd profusely.

But Wayne Newton is not here just to perform. He hopes to win the support of these scientists for a dream he has long held: He wants to exhume Pocahontas. His plan is to reclaim her remains from Gravesend, England, where she is buried, and bring her home to America, and he is here, in Reno, because he has made friends among those of us who may be able to help him do that.

It is possible that no place on earth other than Nevada could have so successfully cultivated a talent such as Wayne Newton's. It is, after all, a place of extreme contrasts: It is the nation's driest state and yet claims the ichthyosaur, an extinct marine reptile, as its state fossil; it is usually classified as a mountain state, despite the fact that most of it lies within the Great Basin; and much of the enormous success of the region has depended for generations on the dismal, often tragic losses of others.

Flying into Reno, you seem to be coming into the center of a piecrust. The crimping at its edges are the Sierra Nevada. The flat center is the Reno-Sparks area. High up, but just under the clouds, the pastry dish appears as a vast, round work of God, or some omniscient baker, whose great desire it was to have man fill the crust with something tempting. Over the years, man has tried to comply.

In the mid-1800s, it seemed that the world itself wanted to travel to Reno. From all over America, people stepped off their porches and into their wagons and moved west. The Donner party was one such group. Tempted by the stories of what lay beyond the mountains, they set out in May 1842 only to get trapped on a Halloween night just southwest of Reno. Of the eighty-seven original members, forty-six lived to tell a tale of terrible survival that included cutting up and roasting the dead for food.

The grisly tale slowed the migration only until the temptation of silver and gold drew thousands of prospectors to the region, providing a westward lure that was unrivaled until 1913, when Nevada became the first state to drop its residency requirement for those seeking divorce to six months. An industry of dude ranches promptly sprang up to house those who were waiting. Then, in 1931, the residency requirement dropped to six weeks, and quickie marriage also became an industry with wedding parlors (no waiting, no blood tests) that continue today to advertise specials such as "love grottoes" and "Roman rooms." In 1971, the world's oldest temptation got a boost with the opening of the Mustang Ranch, which also heralded the legalization of prostitution in twelve of the state's counties.

But amid those lures, as some will tell you, the greatest of all temptations in Reno is the one you can see before you even get off plane. When taxiing down the runway, one sees an airplane hangar emblazoned with THE HIGH ROLLERS, presaging Reno's real draw—slot machines and gambling tables. Gamblers have only to grab their overhead bags and deplane to get a hit. Right outside the arrival gates the games begin, lining the airport corridors as no coffee bar, souvenir shop or shoeshine stand could do.

Cannibalism, prospecting, gambling, prostitution, quickie marriage and divorce: With a past like that, it's a good bet that this is a city perfect for a convention.

A year earlier, the American Academy of Forensic Sciences had chosen Orlando, Florida, for its annual meeting. For a week in the middle of February, the world's leading witnesses for the dead brought tales of murder and mayhem to Tomorrowland and Mickey's Toontown Fair. Some people even brought their kids. Then everyone packed up and went back to real life—the witness stand, the morgue and Court TV—only to meet up again here a year later, in the biggest little city in the world.

As with any convention, there are the reacquaintances. Charging down the vast hall is Neal Haskell, the bug man from Indiana, talking to Laura, the FBI agent who attended his school in May. They are reviewing last-minute details of the poster session she will present of her research into the effects of burnt flesh on the timeline of bug infestation. Haskell is wearing a sports coat that looks as though it comes out of the closet only for weddings and wakes. Laura is sleek in black. They pause for a minute nearby, and then he looks up at me and suggests, "Dinner, tonight. Here. Five-thirty?"

Oh, good, dinner tonight with the bug people—always something to look forward to.

Speaking of food, there's Richard Rosner, medical director of the forensic psychiatry clinic of Bellevue Hospital at the Manhattan District Attorney's office. Easily recognizable, his elasticized suspenders buoy the perimeter of trousers around his circumference, making him look like a man in a barrel—which is appropriate, considering his subspecialty. As founder and president of the Gourmet Club of the American Academy of Forensic Sciences, he indulges in constant research and consultation in the months leading up to the conference, culminating in one great meal to which sixty members are invited at the restaurant of Rosner's exacting choice.

Dr. Rosner has been arranging these meals for nearly twenty years for this group and longer for two other professional groups in his forensic specialty.

Why?

"Consider those people who live in parts of the country where there really are either no restaurants worth speaking about or no wine stores worth speaking about or, alternatively," he says, sighing, "those who, although they are interested in food or wine, have no training and no idea how to order either. We try to remedy this particular social deficiency."

Dr. Rosner also makes himself available for consultation. There were some great meals last year in Orlando, and everyone wants to know where to eat during the week.

"No," he asserts, with a flourish. "You don't come to Reno to eat.

"But next year," he adds, trailing off as if on the track of a scent, "Seattle."

When not eating, a conventioneer's time will be spent at lectures and presentations of academic papers. There's the new stuff—forensic climatology is one of this year's hot topics—as well as the old stuff. The *Proceedings* journal that lists the papers, posters and abstracts is 305 pages long and reads like a *Who's Who* of forensic science. The rest of the time will be spent networking, drinking, gambling, touring the area, showing pictures of the family, exchanging phone numbers with promises to call, and cruising the requisite trade show.

What is hawked, promoted, explained, tested and ultimately bought and sold at trade shows is, of course, the tools of the trade. Here at the trade show for the fifty-second annual AAFS meeting, the booths display new and improved toe tags, rib saws, autopsy tables, DNA collection kits, gloves, soil sifters, microscopes, digital cameras, body-part recovery software, books, knives, scalpels, specimen slides, DNA databasing equipment, spectroscopy systems, lights to make human secretions glow in different colors in the dark, infection-control products, felon-databasing software, consulting services in forensic pathology, toxicology, anthropology and DNA technology, digital evidence documentation stations, spectrum light sources that reveal long-healed bruises beneath the skin from bite marks, fume extractors, metabolic disease–screening technology, imaging and detection devices, genetic identity analysis products, bar code devices for chain-of-evidence integrity, DNA databasing software and hardware, latent fingerprint processing equipment, evidence and property tracking software, postmortem specimen packaging kits and a full range of body bags.

And they give away samples.

While the conference officially begins on Saturday morning, the first few days are mostly for workshops and meetings. For many attendees, the event doesn't really start until the trade show opens on Wednesday morning.

In the nervous moments before the doors open, the people behind the booths can be seen scrambling to lay out their materials and straighten their displays. Outside, most of the attendees gather at the velvet-roped entry, looking very much like the crowd outside Loehmann's on Washington's Birthday. Security guards carefully scrutinize the crowd for the AAFS name tags needed for admission. At the drop of the rope the crowd streams into the exhibit area to see what's new in the technology of crime investigation. The show will be open each day for the remainder of the week from 11 A.M. until 3 P.M. Most people make several trips through.

But for some, the trade show doesn't really happen—meaning that the really good giveaways, the ones kept in cartons under the desks, don't come out—until Henry Lee walks in.

While the average consumer cruising the trade show will pick up latex gloves, pens, pencils, bags (of both the body and book varieties), literature and keychains, when Henry goes shopping, the booth attendants haul out the good stuff: higher-quality T-shirts, stuffed animals, ergonomic squeeze balls in the shapes of various human organs, and whole rolls of neon crime-scene tape. The loot is shoved into his hand and dropped into his bag while salespeople throw their arms over his shoulders, snap his picture and ask him to sign anything they sell. He usually wafts through the trade show with about ten other professionals, but no one gets the same attention as Henry. He is a superstar, and as a result everybody wants him to stretch their brand of fluorescent tape over his crime scenes. Walking in his wake is slow going, but the payoff is terrific.

Hot items at the show this year include the individually wrapped, tiny, single-use saliva alcohol tester (whose manufacturer representative says it is a "real party pleaser"), fingerprinting software CDs and the ergonomic, carpal-tunnel-soothing, squeezable kidney.

Each year the conference has a theme, and this year it is "Truth or Consequences." There will be workshops, poster sessions, papers and presentations held throughout the week on criminalistics, engineering sciences, jurisprudence, odontology, pathology/biology, physical anthropology, psychiatry and behavioral science, questioned documents and toxicology.

Titles of presentations run the gamut from the sublime ("A Comparison of Expirated Bloodstain Patterns with High-Velocity

259

Impact Spatter and Medium-Velocity Impact Spatter Pattern") to the remarkable ("Leave It to Cleaver: Microscopic Analysis of Hacking Trauma on Bone"). Every morning begins with a breakfast seminar with topics and titles varying from year to year, except Friday morning, which is annually reserved for the Tom Krauss Memorial Bite Mark Breakfast. Really.

Most nights there is something going on, as well. Tonight before the scheduled event, though, there is that dinner with the bug people.

Eating with people who love maggots is daunting. At 5:30 sharp, the bug people—yes, there are bug people, just as there are decomp people (although when the groups get together they refer to themselves as the "Maggot-Decomp Gang")—meet at the fancy restaurant on the Nugget's first floor. It's a Mediterranean place with a good wine list and imaginative food.

If there is one piece of advice worth having before sitting down to eat with people who like to talk about maggots over dinner it would simply be: Don't eat rice. But then again, if no one does, Neal Haskell will probably just tell that story again about giving a talk and slide show to an Indiana women's service group when rice was on the menu and showing that picture he has of a face packed with maggot eggs and how many women scurried from the room during the show. It makes him just howl.

Roasted vegetables are not a bad choice, and one would have thought soup was safe at a dinner whose topic will be flesh and bugs.

"Do you know why when young Egyptian princesses died they were not embalmed for several days?" Neal asks no one in particular.

The waitress has just set a bowl in front of the last of the group. She flees. Neal picks up his spoon, which is tiny in his hand.

"To prevent necrophilia," he says happily and dips in.

Haskell has traveled to Reno with three young students—all lovely women in good clothes who are attentive and able to eat right through anything he can toss out—and his attractive, gracious wife, whose dragonfly pin at her shoulder glitters in the candlelight. If not for the subject matter, this could be an extended American family away on vacation.

The news from the farm in Rensselaer is that Neal has a new four-man World War II vehicle he bought from someone in Chicago. Describing himself squeezing into it, he says he is "like a boa trying to get down a sewer pipe," but that he has discovered all kinds of things to shoot out of it, including his new favorite: tennis balls that have been slit open and filled with dirt.

"They'll go half a mile out," he says.

The remainder of dinner is spent discussing how the army is currently experimenting with honeybees, which have an exquisite ability to locate land mines, and how you can attach little microtransmitters to them for the job, as well as Neal's continuing and as yet unrequited quest to get someone to allow him to bring blowflies to a disaster site, say, an airline crash, to home in on the human tissue.

Look at the time. I can't be late to "Bring Your Own Slides," which I host every year on Wednesday night from 7 until 10.

Having signed up in advance, presenters wait their turn in the raucous crowd. Then they eagerly join in a grown-up and professional version of "Show and Tell," offering up and consulting with their peers on their most curious cases.

Consider the so-called "Oddball Case" presented this year by Karen Berka, a scientist in the forensic biology section of the Indiana State Police, Fort Wayne regional laboratory. She has a master's degree from the University of New Haven, where she studied with Henry Lee and learned a thing or two about how to deliver a message.

Berka's case took place in Huntington, Indiana, hometown of Dan Quayle and site of the Dan Quayle Museum, in a home on Route 9, called the Highway of Vice Presidents.

Early in 1999, a caller told local police that a man in town was practicing medicine without a license, a Class D felony. In fact, the man was performing surgery—castrations, to be exact—on willing men who enjoyed extreme body mutilation.

The man performing the surgery stored the excised testes in formalin-filled jars—"medical jars, not Ball jars," noted Berka, dryly—labeled RIGHT and LEFT. She theorized that this was done to avoid "a case of mixed nuts." There were nine of them, hence the "Oddball" moniker Berka had cited.

Testing revealed that the testes "were, in fact, male," and that there were "tons of sample DNA" available, which might be necessary to type participants for trial purposes.

In the course of her fifteen-minute presentation, Berka performed the service not only of raising the spirits of her colleagues but also of informing them about how a freelance body-modification business might look in Hometown, USA. This was new stuff to almost everyone in the room.

The apartment of the man performing the surgeries housed many video tapes of this procedure as well as surgical equipment he had apparently procured from a veterinarian. Despite the surgical supply, however, the evidence suggested that the procedures could take as long as two hours. Berka reminded the audience that to castrate a bull takes somewhere in the neighborhood of 2.5 seconds. The reason for the lengthy procedure was purely commercial: "The money is in the videos" made during the surgery, Berka said. These tapes can be purchased at various castration websites. The so-called surgeon pleaded guilty, got a suspended sentence and moved to Tennessee.

There was a noticeable stream to the bar after those slides.

The history of "Bring Your Own Slides" corresponds to one of the simpler but fundamental advances in the way we investigate crime.

In the early 1960s, while I was still a resident in pathology at Bellevue, Milton Helpern, then the chief medical examiner of New York City, invited me to my first AAFS conference, then held at the Drake Hotel in Chicago. The scene boggled my mind: Until that time I had not realized there were other forensic pathologists with the same enthusiasm and passion I had and, more important, with differing interpretations of how cases should be handled.

I quickly noticed that many of the papers were accompanied by wonderful crime scene photographs taken by the scientists. We didn't do that in New York at that time. All our crime scene photographs were taken by the police. I had a lot to learn about what that meant.

After his paper, Joe Rupp, then chief medical examiner in Fort Lauderdale, invited me to a small, informal meeting of other pathologists. It was held in someone's hotel room and attended by eight medical examiners showing slides, talking and passing a bottle of Jack Daniel's. (I was solemnly instructed that this was not bourbon, but sour mash.) There were paper cups in the bathroom and we drank it neat, since we couldn't afford ice.

The alcohol did nothing to dampen our enthusiasm for curious cases, many of which involved the odd ways people die accidentally. Of particular interest were autoerotic deaths, in which people who create devices to heighten sexual pleasure die when the device malfunctions. Wrong assumptions at these scenes can wreak havoc on an investigation.

Dr. Rupp shared a case in which an elderly fellow was found dead in his bed lying next to a vacuum cleaner. The hose of the device was over the man's penis and contained semen. It took his experience interpreting such scenes to determine that the man had died of a heart attack while masturbating into the suction of the machine.

It was also in this room that I saw the "Love Bug" case, involving an airline pilot in Fort Lauderdale and his Volkswagen. Apparently, the pilot would tie off the steering wheel to set the car to drive in small circles, put the vehicle in gear and then run behind it in a desolate area. He would do so wearing nothing but a homemade metal chain harness that encircled his shoulders and legs and attached to the bumper, and would apparently get sexual pleasure as he chased his car. The last time he did this, the chain attaching him to the bumper got caught around the axle of the rear wheel. Evidence from the scene suggested that as the car went around, it shortened the chain, pulling it taut and crushing him against the Volkswagen.

Imagine being the responding police officer at this scene and trying to determine what had happened. Or the medical examiner at the morgue, seeing only the wounds incurred without having visited the scene or viewed the scene photographs.

Or consider Joe Rupp's case involving a man with a fractured skull found dead in an empty swimming pool.

Did he commit suicide? Was he depressed? Did his wife push him? The police could not make any headway with it until Rupp, who had taken a series of photos at the scene, went back to those photos and observed that one of the man's shoes remained on the pool deck, its long, untied shoelace still attached. That night, during that slide show, we sat amazed and hushed as we realized that the dead man had accidentally tripped over his own shoelace.

Moments of education mingle with entertainment during this particular Wednesday night's "Bring Your Own Slides," and today we pack the largest room at the conference site. Following Karen Berka and the "Oddball" case was Robert Ressler, who profiled serial killers for the FBI. "The bad news/good news here," he said, as the image of two men sharing a meal shined on the screen, "is that I am having lunch with Jeffrey Dahmer."

Participants saw a case of a woman found burned in a fire pit who had consumed such a vast amount of alcohol—an empty tequila bottle and twelve empty beer cans were found at her side—that when she fell in she could not revive. They considered the jurisdictional and identification problems arising when 195 coffins from one county floated into adjoining counties after flooding in North Carolina. They reviewed the case of dental identification on a headless corpse (porcelain crown fragments were found in the stomach). And finally, but not the least of the presentations, there was a rousing game of forensic Jeopardy.

With the names LEE, BILL and WAYNE printed on placards before them, the contestants battled amid the categories "Forensic People," "Things That Bite," "Things That Suck," "Things That Stick," "Things That Rot" and "Digging Things Up."

Category: Forensic People for three hundred.

Answer: The man who says that pubic lice is every entomologist's best friend.

Question: Who is Wayne Lord of the FBI, otherwise known as Lord of the Flies?

It was a rough night.

During the days there is a lot of dropping in and out of talks—catch a little update on crime scene technology and then you might be ready for a discussion of the ethics of dealing with expert witnesses. After an hour of odontology, it might make sense to listen to a gunshot wound update.

Some of this requires making hard choices. There were seven competing concurrent presentations about deaths associated with liposuction. There were four on the epidemiology of serial homicide. On Thursday afternoon there were offerings in all thirteen conference rooms (the names of which include Bonanza, Ponderosa and South Pacific).

Meanwhile, the physical anthropology session in Bonanza B was standing room only during two talks on the whereabouts of Russian Grand Duchess Anastasia. Professionals who usually dip in and out of these lectures—interested, of course, but rarely to the point of waiting in line—stood patiently to get into this talk. And then they crammed the hall so that it was hot, airless and absolutely packed.

The first presenter in the session was the Russian scientist Sergei Alekseevich Nikitin of Moscow. Speaking in Russian with a simultaneous English translator, he explained that his identifications were based primarily on the photographic superimposition of the reconstructed skulls on early photographs of the Romanov girls.

By 1992, he said, Russian experts had used the photo-superimposition method—literally, one photograph laid over another—to determine that the remains of the nine skeletons were those of Tsar Nicholas II; Tsarina Alexandra Feodorovna; their daughters Olga, Tatiana (skeleton #5) and Anastasia (skeleton #6); Dr. Botkin; the butler, Troup; the chambermaid, Demidova; and the cook, Kharitonov.

Photos of the girls taken in May 1917 were shown on the screen at the front of the room. One reveals Grand Duchess Marie standing next to a soldier holding an S. Mosin infantry rifle, a weapon whose height, with bayonet, is approximately 170 centimeters. Nikitin explained that this value was then compared with the heights of Tatiana and Anastasia. Next the femur bones of the girls were measured. From this measurement, the height of skeleton #5 was determined to be 165–170 centimeters, while #6 was 160–165 centimeters. In 1994, using the skulls that were found, the faces of the deceased were reconstructed.

As he spoke, Dr. Nikitin produced a chilling gift for the AAFS collection: a smooth plaster head that he said had been rendered from the facial reconstruction of Anastasia's skull. A hush fell over the packed house as the beautiful face topping a long, slender neck passed from hand to hand, its blank eyes looking out to us, seeming to take in the crowd, as if to make a mute expert witness corroboration to the staunch belief of Dr. Nikitin that Anastasia had, indeed, been laid to rest.

But then the microphone was passed to physical anthropologist Dr. Diane France of the Laboratory for Human Identification at Colorado State University, who presented her findings, which agreed with those of the Maples team I was on with Lowell Levine: The remains of Anastasia had yet to be found.

No slugfest, no arguments, no international debate; just science versus science, as it is every single day in this business.

All week long, choices have to be made among such compelling and competing topics as serial killer profiling, injury patterns, fingerprinting, hair and fiber analysis, Santeria and ritualistic writing, ballpoint pen ink analysis, drug use among tractor-trailer drivers, con men, DNA, digital analysis of bite marks, ballistics, death by a bangstick shark gun, forensic nursing, the aging of dried blood spots, DNA plant typing, finding fingerprints on crack cocaine, a suicide in New Jersey in which a man encased his whole body in a rubber suit and rebreather, self-inflicted stab wounds, kids in court, and the possible exhumation of George Washington to answer paternity questions.

Oh yes, somewhere between breakfasts, lectures, lunches, posters, dinners and the trade show, I met with Henry Lee and Wayne Newton to talk about the Pocahontas project. Newton seems sincere. His Native-American ancestry includes Pocahontas's Powhatan tribe, and he thinks that more than 380 years in English soil is long enough, that it's time to bring Pocahontas home and bury her in her native Virginia. Henry is on board. So am I.

By the end of the week, the requisite roll of quarters you've been carrying with you everywhere starts to look and feel like a weapon. Tightly wrapped in orange-and-white waxed paper that says LEAVE NOTHING TO CHANCE, it has started to feel good in the fist. But, then, even the slits in the stainless steel toiletry vending machines in the bathrooms have started to look like slots that might yield a big win from those quarters. And there's the cold, hard fact that daylight in Reno has been replaced by neon.

It's time to get out of town.

Acknowledgments

Together we would like to thank our agent, Kristine Dahl, for challenging us to find a new voice in which to tell this story, for knowing exactly what to say each time we came to her (especially that she hides under her bedcovers to read true crime books) and for her contagious sense of wonder and enthusiasm. We wish to thank David Rosenthal, our publisher at Simon & Schuster, for having faith and getting the concept from the start, and Bob Bender, our editor, for his consummate skill and cool but firm hand in guiding the project.

We are grateful to Jeff Cohen, of the Albany *Times Union*, for introducing us, buying dinner and then sitting back and letting us start this conversation.

Many professionals in the forensic sciences gave their time and attention and opened their labs and homes to us. We particularly want to thank Dr. Henry Lee, his wife, Margaret, Dr. Lowell Levine, Dr. Neal Haskell and Dr. Herbert Leon MacDonell for

letting Marion come and have a good look. Our thanks go to
Major Timothy McAuliffe and Lt. Kevin Costello, both of the
New York State Police, for everything, including their patience,
friendship and, of course, diet tips. And thanks to New York State
Police Superintendent William McMahon for his support. We are
grateful to Virginia Lynch, a constant source of inspiration to all
who know her. We want to acknowledge Judge Haskell Pitluck
for all the answers to all the questions we could think of, and
Enrico Togneri, for answering all the ones we didn't think to
ask—as well as for the tour of Reno. Special Agent Terrence
Thomas of the Florida Department of Law Enforcement was gen-
erous with his time and attention, as was Karen Berka, of the Indiana State Police. We are also grateful to Dr. Cyril Wecht, Dr.
Werner Spitz, Dr. L.J. Dragovic, Professor James Starrs, Robert
Hazelwood, Dr. Marie Russell, Dr. Richard Rosner, Dr. Ira Titu-
nik, Brian Gestring, Dr. Fred Rieders, Bob Ford, Abdul Salam,
George Castelle, Dr. James Young, Herb Buckley, Greg Welch,
Johanna Li and Suzanne Anderson.

Michael is grateful to my wife, Linda B. Kenney, my brother,
Robert, and my children, Dr. Trissa A. Baden, Dr. Lindsey R.
Baden and Sarah D. Baden, for their love and encouragement in
all my endeavors. I work with the integrity and honesty of my late
son, Jud Baden, always close to my heart. My thanks go to Pat
Hulbert for all the things she does. I thank Marion for wanting to
do this book and for putting up with me, and I am grateful to her
husband, Rex, for his time, concern and valuable suggestions.

Marion thanks Michael for allowing me into the world he
inhabits and for being brave and trusting enough in another writer
to let this book evolve as it has. My loving and delightful friend
Richard Young deserves all the thanks I can give him for everything he does, as do the other kind inhabitants of Van Hornesville,
New York, where writing is as much a part of its history as the late
August square dance at the Home Farm. To Dr. David Kaplan,
who offered me the skills to be delighted again. My friends Sharon

and Paul get thanks for listening to drafts of this and for sharing their own art with me. Elizabeth called at all the right moments. Thanks to my sweet friend Susannah McCorkle, jazz artist and writer, for singing "The Waters of March" every time it was needed. Kyle was there when the deal was made, and Annie, Nicky, Jane, Debra and Tom literally showed up on the doorstep during the writing with supplies and love. Mary Elizabeth and Mary and Paul made me laugh when I thought I had lost my sense of humor. The evolution of this book is enormously tied to several specific writers and editors I know, foremost among them my sister and friend, Margaret Roach, the boss, whose perfect pitch astonishes all of us; Sydney Schanberg, who urged me to do this just this way (and who has outfitted me with jokes for twenty-five years), and his beautiful wife, Jane Freiman, who asked me to write for her at just the right time; Art Silverman of National Public Radio for his fine ears; the novelist Benjamin Cheever, who read some of the early pages and generously handed over the whip; Gary Taubes, whose voluminous integrity gets him into trouble every time out; and the writers in my classes at the Arts Center of the Capital Region, who teach me more than I teach them. But my deepest gratitude goes to Rex William Smith, the finest newspaperman I have ever known, South Dakota's greatest export, my husband and best friend, who has had his mind changed about many things since I've known him but, apparently, not about me.

Sources

Much of the material in this book comes from the personal experiences of the authors, most notably the twenty thousand autopsies performed and countless investigations undertaken by Dr. Michael Baden during four decades of practice of medical pathology. In addition, Marion Roach interviewed at length some of the experts profiled in this book. Standard references, notably *Gray's Anatomy*, were invaluable in interpreting medical and scientific matters. In certain cases, court papers and law enforcement documents were reviewed for background as well as explanation of specific events. The authors wish to acknowledge their debt to the scientists and writers whose publications are cited below, while accepting for themselves full responsibility for the accuracy and completeness of the citations.

Articles, Reports and Miscellaneous Sources

Altimari, David. "The Search for Pocahontas Includes Some Famous Names." *Hartford Courant,* March 30, 2000.

Berlow, Alan. "The Wrong Man." *The Atlantic Monthly,* November 1999.

Bunyan, Nigel. "Killer Trapped by Prints of His Ears." *The Daily Telegraph,* December 16, 1998.

Burns, Ric. "The Donner Party." Documentary created for the *American Experience* series on Public Broadcasting Service, 1992.

Castelle, George. "Lab Fraud: Lessons Learned." *The Champion,* National Association of Criminal Defense Lawyers, May 1999.

"The Dead Rise Again in the Courtroom." *The National Law Journal,* June 21, 1993.

Gillman, Todd J. "Death Penalty Under Scrutiny from All Sides." *Dallas Morning News,* July 11, 2000.

Hanna, Bill. "Relatives Upset Over Exhumed Body; In a Search for Jesse James, the Wrong Body Was Dug Up at Granbury Cemetery." *Fort Worth Star-Telegram,* August 19, 2000.

Hansen, Mark. "Experts to Go." *ABA Journal,* February 2000.

Lewis, Neil A. "Study Finds Strong Evidence Jefferson Fathered Slave Son." *New York Times,* January 27, 2000.

MacDonald, Elizabeth. "The Making of an Expert Witness: It's in the Credentials." *Wall Street Journal,* February 8, 1999.

"Mass Spectronomy." *The Salt Lake Tribune,* October 9, 1997.

McCormick, John. "Software, Scene of the Crime." *Newsweek,* February 28, 2000.

McGrew, Janell. "Justice Denied: The Willie Edwards Story." *Montgomery Advertiser,* January 23–28, 2000.

Messina, Larence. "Court Asked to Review Zain Report." *Charleston (W. Va.) Gazette,* June 2, 1999.

Nawrocki, Stephen P., Ph.D. Instructional materials prepared for the Forensic Entomology and Anthropology Field Training Workshop in Rensselaer, Indiana, June 2–3, 1999.

Nieves, Evelyn. "In a Booming Reno, No Room for the Old Inn." *New York Times,* January 25, 2000.

Pavich, Robert M. "Hoffa." *Detroit News,* July 31, 1995.

Poole, Jenny. "Forensic Facial Reconstruction Released in Effort to ID Victims." *Chattanooga Times Free Press,* April 20, 2000.

Posner, Gerald. "A Murder in Alabama." *Talk,* June 2000.

Prendergast, Jane. "What Science Hopes to Learn by Exhuming Zachary Taylor." *The Cincinnati Enquirer,* June 17, 1991.

"Quietly, DNA Testing Transforms Sleuth's Job." *The New York Times,* March 9, 1999.

Sources

Reynolds, Barbara. "Clues from the Grave." *USA Today,* June 19, 1991.

Ripley, Amanda. "Bone Hunter." *City Paper (D.C.),* March 3, 1998.

Sachs, Jessica Snyder. "A Maggot for the Prosecution." *Discover,* November 1998.

Starrs, James E., and Charles R. Midkiff, senior eds. "Beware Experts—You May Be Next." *Scientific Sleuthing Review, The Many Uses of the Forensic Sciences* 22, no. 4, Winter 1998.

U.S. Department of Justice. *Convicted by Juries, Exonerated by Science.* Washington, D.C., June 1996.

Van der Lugt, Cor. "Ear Identification: State of the Art." Paper presented at the conference for shoe print and toolmark examiners, Noordwijkerhout, Neth., April 24, 1997.

Wade, Nicholas. "After Jefferson, a Question About Washington and a Young Slave." *The New York Times,* July 7, 1999.

Walt, Kathy. "Debate over Death Penalty Is Renewed." *Houston Chronicle,* July 9, 2000.

Watson, Andrew. "New Tools: A New Breed of High-Tech Detectives." *Science* 289, no. 5481, August 2000.

"Way in Which Public Defenders are Chosen in the State of Texas." National Public Radio, morning edition, July 13, 2000. Anchor: Madeleine Brand; reporter: Janet Heimlich.

"Whose Body of Evidence?" *The Economist* 348, July 1, 1998.

Books

Bailey, F. Lee, with Harvey Aronson. *The Defense Never Rests.* New York: Penguin Books, 1971.

Catts, E. Paul, and Neal H. Haskell. *Entomology & Death: A Procedural Guide.* Clemson, S.C.: Joyce's Print Shop, 1990.

Cooper, Cynthia L., and Sam Reese Sheppard. *Mockery of Justice: The True Story of the Sheppard Murder Case.* New York: Penguin Books, 1995.

Dumas, Timothy. *A Wealth of Evil: The True Story of the Murder of Martha Moxley in America's Richest Community.* New York: Warner Books, 1998.

Evans, Colin. *The Casebook of Forensic Detection: How Science Solved 100 of the World's Most Baffling Crimes.* New York: John Wiley & Sons, 1996.

Firstman, Richard, and Jamie Talan. *The Death of Innocents.* New York: Bantam Books, 1997.

Frisbie, Thomas, and Randy Garrett. *Victims of Justice.* New York: Avon Books, 1998.

Fuhrman, Mark. *Murder in Greenwich: Who Killed Martha Moxley?* New York: HarperCollins, 1998.

Sources

Goff, M. Lee, Amy Bartlett Wright, illustrator. *A Fly for the Prosecution: How Insect Evidence Helps Solve Crimes.* Cambridge, Mass.: Harvard University Press, 2000.

Hickey, Charles, Todd Lightly, and John O'Brien. *Goodbye, My Little Ones: The True Story of a Murderous Mother and Five Innocent Victims.* New York: Penguin Books, 1996.

Houde, John. *Crime Lab: A Guide for Nonscientists.* Ventura, Calif.: Calico Press, 1999.

Joyce, Christopher, and Eric Stover. *Witnesses from the Grave: The Stories Bones Tell.* New York: Ballantine Books, 1991.

Lee, Dr. Henry, and Dr. Jerry Labriola. *Famous Crimes Revisited.* Southington, Conn.: Strong Books, 2001.

Lewis, Alfred Allan, with Herbert Leon MacDonell. *The Evidence Never Lies: The Casebook of a Modern Sherlock Holmes.* New York: Dell Publishing, 1984.

Maples, William R., Ph.D., and Michael Browning. *Dead Men Do Tell Tales: The Strange and Fascinating Cases of a Forensic Anthropologist.* New York: Doubleday, 1994.

McAlary, Mike. *Cop Shot: The True Story of a Murder That Shocked the Nation.* New York: G.P. Putnam's Sons, 1990.

McGinnis, Joe. *Blind Faith.* New York: Penguin Books, 1989.

McPhee, John. *Irons in the Fire.* New York: Farrar, Straus and Giroux, 1997.

Michaud, Stephen G., with Roy Hazelwood. *The Evil That Men Do.* New York: St. Martin's Press, 1998.

Nickell, Joe, and John F. Fischer. *Crime Science: Methods of Forensic Detection.* Lexington, Ky.: The University Press of Kentucky, 1999.

Ragle, Larry. *Crime Scene.* New York: Avon Books, 1995.

Rule, Ann. *Bitter Harvest: A Woman's Fury, A Mother's Sacrifice.* New York: Simon & Schuster, 1997.

Scheck, Barry, Peter Neufeld, Jim Dwyer. *Actual Innocence: Five Days to Execution and other Dispatches from the Wrongfully Convicted.* New York: Doubleday, 2000.

Sereny, Gitta. *The Invisible Children: Child Prostitution in America, West Germany and Great Britain.* New York: Alfred A. Knopf, 1995.

Simon, David. *Homicide: A Year on the Killing Streets.* New York: Houghton Mifflin, 1991.

Spitz, Werner U., and Russell S. Fisher. *Medicolegal Investigation of Death.* Springfield, Ill.: Charles C. Thomas, 1993.

Starr, Douglas. *Blood: An Epic History of Medicine and Commerce.* New York: Alfred A. Knopf, 1998.

Wecht, Cyril, M.D., J.D., with Mark Curriden and Benjamin Wecht. *Cause of Death.* New York: Penguin Books, 1993.

———. *Grave Secrets.* New York: Penguin Books, 1996.

Sources

Wilcox, Robert K. *The Mysterious Deaths at Ann Arbor.* Terre Haute, Ind.: Popular Library, 1977.
Zonderman, Jon. *Beyond the Crime Lab: The New Science of Investigation.* New York: John Wiley & Sons, 1999.

Websites

Berry, Sheila Martin. "When Experts Lie."
www.truthinjustice.org/expertslie.htm [March 14, 2001].
Cruickshank, Douglas. "Last Roundup at the Mustang Ranch."
www.salon.com/people/rogue/1999/08/12/mustang/index.html [March 14, 2001].
"Ear Print Catches Murderer."
http://news.bbc.co.uk/hi/english/uk/newsid_235000/235721.stm#top [March 20, 2001].
Horton, Gary A. "A Water History of Nevada."
www.state.nv.us/cnr/ndwp/history/nevada.htm [March 14, 2001].
"Judge Clears Photographers Implicated in Diana Crash."
www.cnn.com/world/europe/9909/03/france.diana/index.html [March 20, 2001].
Neville, Wesley. "Forensic Art: Little Known—Highly Effective."
www.forensicartist.com/article.html [March 14, 2001].
"Unknown Soldier's Exhumation Begins."
www.arlingtoncemetery.com/unk-vn31.htm [March 20, 2001].
Website of the medical examiner of Hamilton County, Tennessee:
www.hamiltontn.gov/medicalexaminer/DEFAULT.HTM [March 20, 2001].
Woodhouse, Leighton. "Who Killed Meriwether Lewis?"
www.salon.com/it/feature/1999/03/22 feature.html [March 20, 2001].

Index

abdominal wall, 103, 104
abuse, 169, 171
accidental deaths, 75, 100, 209
    airline disasters and, 61–62, 214, 261
    autoerotic, 263–64
    see also auto accidents
Adams, Randall Dale, 242–43
adipocere, 183
admissibility of evidence, 80–82
    expert testimony and, *see* qualifying
        process
age, 104, 210, 211, 221
airline disasters, 61–62, 214, 261
Albert, Marv, 214
alcohol, 19, 41, 106, 264
    Diana's death and, 215, 217–18
alcoholism, 109, 217
Alexandra Feodorovna, Tsarina, 182,
    183, 184, 266
algor mortis, 19, 20
Alien Autopsy: Fact or Fiction, 91
American Academy of Forensic Sciences
    (AAFS), Reno convention of,
    253–67
American College of Forensic Examiners
    (ACFE), 244–45

Anastasia, Grand Duchess of Russia,
    182, 183, 185, 265–66
anatomical quirks, 105
anatomic pathology, 80
anchor points, 221
Anderson, Anna, 182, 185
animals, 103, 211, 216
anthropology, forensic, 183, 211–12,
    265–66
ants, 170–71
appendix, 109–10
Argentina, "disappeared ones" in, 214
Arlington National Cemetery, 188–89, 194
arms, 113
arrests, wrongful, 247
arsenic, 190, 219–20
arteriosclerosis, 107–8
artificial intelligence, 146
artists, forensic, 209, 220–24
asphyxiation, *see* suffocation
assistant district attorneys (ADAs), 15,
    17, 111–12
assumptions, incorrect, 263
    in Binion case, 62–64, 67–79
    forensic animation software and,
        245–46

Index

atlas, 210
attorneys:
    ADAs, 15, 17, 111–12
    logical sequence of questions from, 80
    in preparation of expert testimony,
        79–80
    see also defense; prosecution
auto accidents, 99, 106, 245
    insects and, 163, 171
    "Love Bug" case and, 263–64
    of Princess Diana, 215–18
autoerotic deaths, 263–64
autopsies, 15–32, 80
    attire for, 18
    checking that body is dead in, 23
    collecting samples in, 27–30, 106–7
    comparing body to driver's license
        photo in, 23, 24
    cost of, 98–99
    courtroom testimony about, 83,
        87–88, 195–96
    cutting oneself during, 96, 97, 110
    cutting through rib cage in, 104
    decision to proceed with, 97–98, 140,
        189
    doing only what is needed in, 113, 115
    on exhumed remains, 193–98,
        200–203
    external examination in, 26–27,
        30–32, 117
    facts accompanying body in, 24–26,
        101
    faked by Erdmann, 239–41
    fingerprinting in, 26, 115
    incisions in, 95–97, 111
    internal examination in, 95–118
    organs examined in, 103, 105–13
    photographs in, 24, 28–29, 115–16
    re-autopsy and, 65
    respect for human body in, 97,
        101–2, 115–16, 209
    restoration of body after, 117–18
    tape recording notes during, 26,
        116–17
    thoroughness required in, 102
    tissue samples in, 71
    tools for, 14, 95–96, 102–3, 104
    uniqueness of each body in, 104–5
    visual inspection in, 26–27, 30–32
    see also homicide autopsies
Autopsy, 200
autopsy reports, 118
    falsified, 239–41
    notes for, 26, 116–17
autopsy suites, 14

autopsy tables, 14, 17
Avdonin, Alexander, 182–83

babies, misidentification of, 22–23
Bacon, Sir Francis, 186, 231
Ballard, Norman, 241
ballistics, 81–82
    blood loss and, 40
Balonis, Kathie, 235
barbiturates, 19
Barshop, Steven, 142
Bass, William, 164
bear paws, 62
Beckwith, Byron De La, 192–93,
    195–96
bees, 163, 171, 261
beetles, 170, 173
Bellevue Psychiatric Hospital, 137–38
Belushi, John, 91
Berka, Karen, 261–62
Bertillon system, 224
Binion, Lonnie Ted:
    author's expert testimony on death of,
        83–92
    author's findings on death of, 67–79
    incorrectly assumed to be suicide,
        62–64
    preliminary hearing on death of, 70,
        76, 78, 84–88, 89
    trial for murder of, 88–92
bite marks, 213, 214
Black Panther case, 37
bland hemorrhage, 72
Blassie, Michael J., 188–89
Bleak House (Dickens), 127
blood, 26
    in autopsies, 17, 95–96, 106
    bruises and, 72
    circulation of, 39–40, 70, 73, 107
    constituents of, 40
    at crime scenes, protection of,
        149–50
    DNA in, 145, 164, 172, 197
    individual drops of, 45–48
    insects and, 171, 172
    MacDonell's training sessions on,
        36–56
    spraying from nose and mouth,
        53–56
    surface tension and, 40–41
    Zain's junk science and, 229–31,
        235–39
blood alcohol concentration (BAC), 41,
    215, 217–18
blood pattern analysis, 36–56

experiments and, 38–39, 41–45,
  48–50, 53–56
gunshots and, 51–53
Mowbray case and, 50–53
Simpson case and, 45–48
blowflies, 163, 170, 171, 261
board certification, 243–45
bodies:
  absence of, 60–62, 124–25
  changes in, after death, 19–20
  headless, 264–65
  identification of, *see* identification
  live, in morgue, 23
  mixed up, 22–23
  moved after death, 32, 169
  respect for, 97, 101–2, 115–16, 209
  see also autopsies; homicide autopsies
body bags, 13–14
  insect evidence in, 168
  removing body from, 20
  search of, 20
  unzipping of, 17, 18
Body Farm, 164–65
body fluids, autopsy table design and, 17
body lice, 171, 172, 265
body temperature, after death, 19–20,
  150
Bonaventure, Joseph, 92
bone fragments, 125
bones, 183, 184
  age of, 211
  in head and face, 210
  skeletonized remains and, 210,
    211–12
booties:
  for autopsies, 18
  for crime scenes, 149, 150
Boston Strangler, 196–98
Bradford, Ricky, 240
Brady rule, 77
brain, 106, 209, 210
  examination of, 112–13
braincase, 210
Brando, Cheyenne, 141
Brando, Christian, 141–43
Brando, Marlon, 141–43
Breathalyzer, 38
Britt, Raymond C., 199, 200
Britton, Albert, 192
Brooks, Ellen, 201, 202–3
bruises, 112–13, 213
  in Binion case, 71–72, 73, 76, 78
  from CPR, 72, 73
  natural sequence of, 71–72
buccal cells, 197

bugs, *see* insects
Bundy, Ted, 214
burden of proof, 153
burials, 102
  coffins moved by flood waters and,
    264
  illicit, 190
  wrong bodies in graves and, 22, 23
  see also exhumations
Burke, William, 76
burking, 76–77, 85

calcium, 211
carbon monoxide poisoning, 32, 103
cardiopulmonary resuscitation (CPR), 72,
  73
cartilage, 104
caskets, 191
Castelle, George, 248
castrations, 262
cause of death, 16, 59–61
  incorrect assumptions about, 62–64,
    67–79
  never determined, 60–61
cement liners, for coffins, 191
Centers for Disease Control (CDC),
  234–35
cervix, 110
Chambers, Robert, 131
chasing the dragon, 68, 75, 85
Chattanooga Times Free Press, 223–24
Chicago Tribune, 247
child abuse, 169, 171
cigarette butts, 197
circulatory system, 39–40, 70, 73, 107
Cisneros, Aureliano, 162–63, 168
civil cases, 82
  insurance claims and, 66–67
Clark, Marcia, 149
climatology, forensic, 257
clinical pathology, 80
Clinton, Bill, 132
clothes, 27
  from crime scene, 22
  insect evidence in, 168
  removing from body, 29
  searching for semen on, 26, 30
cockroaches, 171
coffins, 191, 192, 264
Cohen, William, 189
collateral attacks, 90–92
collecting samples, 27–30, 106–7
confessions, 64, 145, 153, 172
Congress, U.S., 91, 193
Connally, John, 20

Index

Connecticut State Police Crime Lab,
    129–31
contingency fees, 66, 67
convictions, wrongful, *see* wrongful con-
    victions
coroners, 98, 100, 234–35
court proceedings, 16, 21
    autopsy reports and, 26
    civil *vs.* criminal, 66–67
    exhumations and, 195–96
    experts' testimony in, 79–92; *see also*
        expert witnesses
    forensic entomology and, 165–66, 168
    preparing to testify in, 79–80
    testimony about autopsies in, 83,
        87–88, 195–96
    see also judges; juries; preliminary
        hearings
Court TV, 91
Crafts, Helle and Richard, 123–26
cranium, 210
Crater, Joseph E., 60
credentialing process, 243–45
cremation, 182, 184
crime lab, birth of, 126–27
crime scenes, 85, 130, 133, 140–53
    blood pattern analysis and, 36–56
    bloody, cockroach tracks in, 171
    communication between autopsy
        suite and, 16–17, 29, 113
    establishing perimeter at, 148–49
    first hour of, 148
    first person arriving at, 148
    medical examiner's prompt arrival at,
        150–52
    never rushing to body at, 170
    photographs of, 28–29, 46, 48, 152,
        263
    police disruption of evidence at, 26,
        46–48, 63, 148–53
    police sent to, 59, 63, 64
    protecting and collecting evidence at,
        21, 25–26, 29, 63, 64, 100, 101,
        140, 142–43, 145, 146, 148–53
    removing body from, 46–47, 152
    in Simpson case, 140, 148–53
    trace evidence at, 21, 29, 63, 64,
        144–46, 148–53
criminalistics, 122–34
    birth of modern crime lab and,
        126–27
    defined, 21
criminal trials, 82
    lack of expert witnesses in, 67
crowners, 100

cutting onself during autopsy, 96, 97, 110
cyanide, 18–19

Dahmer, Jeffrey, 264
d'Arbois, Bergeret, 159
Daubert rule, 81–82, 165–66, 234, 243
Davis, Dewey, 238
Davis, Gerald Wayne, 238
Davis, Jack, 235
dead person, respect for, 97, 101–2, 115,
    209
death, 139
    body changes after, 19–20
    cause and manner of, 59–61, 75,
        201–2; *see also* cause of death;
        manner of death
    insects attracted by, 159
    place of, 32, 169
    scenes of, 138–40; *see also* crime
        scenes
    smell of, 18, 159, 171
    time of, *see* time of death
    way of life reflected in, 19, 104, 105
death certificates, 97–98, 117
    issued without body, 61–62
death penalty, 67, 78
    junk science and, 234, 237, 239,
        241–43
    quality of legal counsel and, 247,
        248–49
    in Texas, 241–43, 248–49
decomposition, 14, 18, 27, 113, 114–15,
    207
    five major stages of, 170
    lab devoted to study of, 164–65
defense, 233
    degree of guilt and, 77–78
    prosecution findings revealed to, 77,
        108
    quality of, in capital cases, 247,
        248–49
degree of guilt, 77–78
degrees of proof, 84
DeLaughter, Bobby, 193, 194
dental work, *see* teeth and dental work
dentistry, forensic, 113, 114, 183,
    212–15
DeSalvo, Albert, 196
detectives, 140
    at autopsies, 15–16, 17, 23, 24–26,
        111–13
    at crime scenes, 63, 64
    see also police
de Vere, Edward, 186
Diana, Princess of Wales, 106, 215–18

Dickens, Charles, 127
dieners, 15, 17
Dillard, Tom, 67–70, 75–78, 85, 90
DiMaio, Vincent, 238
disappearances, 60–61, 62
    Crafts case and, 123–26
disclosure of evidence, 77, 108
discoloration, lividity and, 19, 20, 32,
    40, 47, 150
disinterment, see exhumations
dismemberment, 209
DNA, 27, 29, 62, 132, 144–46, 153,
    164, 181, 197, 216, 246, 249,
    262
    exhumations and, 184–85, 187, 188,
        189
    extracted from insects, 171, 172
    identifications made from, 144–46,
        184–85, 207, 212
    juries influenced by, 146
    in overturning of wrongful convic-
        tions, 230–31, 237, 238, 247
    Romanovs' remains and, 184–85
DNA fingerprinting, 144
DNA testing, 144–45
Donner party, 255
Doyle, Sir Arthur Conan, 126–27
driver's licenses, 23, 24
Drollet, Dag, 141–43
drowning, 201
drugs, 31, 106–7, 171
    body changes after death and, 20
    hair testing for, 215, 216–17, 218
    interaction of, 75
dusting for prints, 38

ear prints, 224
ears, 104, 208, 210, 221
Edwards, Malinda, 200–201, 202
Edwards, Willie, 198–203
Egypt, ancient, 260
Einstein, Albert, 232
embalming, 47, 104, 260
emergency rooms, 22, 25
emotionally disturbed people, 105
entomology, forensic, 158–76, 265
    see also insects
Erdmann, Ralph, 239–41
erection, strangulation and, 28
estrogen, 110
ethanol, 19
ethics tests, for board certification,
    244–45
Evers, Medgar, 192–96, 200
Evers, Van, 194–95

evidence:
    admissibility of, 80–82; see also quali-
        fying process
    at crime scene, protecting and collect-
        ing of, 21, 25–26, 29, 63, 64,
        100, 101, 140, 142–43, 145, 146,
        148–53
    criminalistics and, 123
    disclosure of, to other side, 77, 108
    falsification of, 229–31, 232–33,
        235–41, 247
    police disruption of, 26, 46–48, 63,
        148–53
    see also trace evidence
Evidence Never Lies, The (MacDonell),
    81
exhumations, 180–203, 212
    Boston Strangler and, 196–98
    Edwards case and, 198–203
    Erdmann's faked autopsies and,
        239–41
    to establish paternity, 186–88
    Evers case and, 192–96, 200
    family members and, 189, 192, 194
    of manuscripts, 185–86
    new questions raised by, 196–98
    to perform autopsy, 193–98,
        200–203
    of Pocahontas, 254–55, 267
    of presidents, 187–88
    process of, 190–92
    of Romanov family, 180, 181–85,
        265–66
    of unknown soldier, 188–89
expert witnesses, 48, 66–92, 248
    attacks on credibility of, 90–92
    bias in, 89–90, 91
    Binion case and, 62–64, 67–69,
        83–92
    in civil vs. criminal cases, 66–67
    credentialing process for, 243–45
    junk science and, 229–49
    jury instructed on, 82, 84
    level of communication of, 87
    logical sequence of questions to, 80
    payment of, 83
    preparing to testify, 79–80
    qualifying of, 79–82, 165–66, 234,
        243
    rarely called to witness stand, 69
    speaking to jury, 86
    testifying in court, 79–92
eyeglasses, 221, 222
eyes, 106–7, 208, 210, 221
eyewitnesses, 146

Index

face, 47, 208, 210, 211
  slippage in, 27
facial reconstruction, 113, 209, 220–24,
  266
  two-dimensional (sketches), 222–24
fact testimony, 82–83
Faerstein, Saul, 146–47
fainting, during autopsies, 17
false convictions, *see* wrongful convictions
family:
  autopsies and, 97, 98–99, 102
  exhumations and, 189, 192, 194
  homicides and, 143
  identification of loved one's body by,
    23, 222
  right of, to review medical examiner's
    work, 74
fat, 103–4, 183
Fayed, Dodi Al, 215–18
FBI (Federal Bureau of Investigation),
    114–15, 127, 164, 173, 187, 200,
    203, 247, 264
Federal Occupational Safety and Health
    Administration (OSHA), 18
feet, bags protecting evidence on, 20–21,
    26
Feynman, Richard, 232, 240
fibers, 16, 27, 28, 125
fingernail scrapings, 26
fingerprints, 26, 38, 114–15, 146, 224
fire ants, 170–71
flies, 163, 170, 171, 261
fluorescence, 26, 30
fontanelles, 210
Ford, Robert, 52
Ford, West, 187
forensic animation software, 245–47
forensic anthropology, 183, 211–12,
    265–66
forensic artists, 209, 220–24
forensic climatology, 257
forensic entomology, 158–76, 265
  see also insects
forensic odontology (dentistry), 113,
    114, 183, 212–15
forensic pathology, 80, 83, 99, 100, 140,
    235, 263
  author's beliefs and, 180–81
  birth of modern crime lab and,
    126–27
  history of, 99–100
  occupational hazards of, 96–97
forensic science, 21, 28, 140, 143,
    152–53, 159, 200, 225
  bad practitioners of, 229–31,
    232–49; *see also* junk science

credentialing process in, 243–45
Lee's model crime lab and, 129–31
Reno convention and, 253–67
trade shows and, 258–59
  see also specific fields
Foster, Vincent, 132
France, Diane, 266
Frankfurt plane, 220–21, 223
Frye rule, 81
Fugitive, The, 246
Fuhrman, Mark, 150
funeral directors, 14–15, 22, 47
funeral parlors, 28, 192
future violence, predictions of, 242–43

Gagliardi, Ralph, 114–15
gasoline, 19, 182
genes, 144
genomic (nuclear) DNA, 184, 197, 210
Gilchrist, Joyce, 237
gloves:
  for autopsies, 18, 96
  in protection of crime scenes, 149
Goldman, Ronald, 45–46, 92, 146, 150,
    152
  see also Simpson case
Gorky Park, 209
grand juries, 82
graves, *see* burials; exhumations
Grigson, James, 242
ground penetrating radar (GPR), 190–91
gunshots, 106, 113
  autopsies on exhumed remains and,
    193, 195–96
  blood pattern analysis and, 51–53
  blood spraying from nose and mouth
    compared to, 53–56
  Brando case and, 141–43
  falling down after, 142–43
  wound shape and, 51

hair, 125, 149, 208, 210, 215–20, 222
  anatomy of, 216
  collected during autopsies, 27, 28
  DNA analysis and, 145, 184, 187
  in drug testing, 215, 216–17, 218
  Napoleon's death and, 218–20
  race and, 216
  visual analysis of, 215–16
hairnets, 149
Halloween, 19
handcuff marks, 71, 90
hands, 62
  bags protecting evidence on, 20–21,
    26, 152
Hare, William, 76

Harris, Jean, 37
Harris, William, 236–37
Haskell, Chrissy, 165
Haskell, Jane, 174, 261
Haskell, Neal, 158–75, 256–57, 260–61
    Cisneros case and, 162–63, 168
head, 208–25
    bones in, 210
    cleaning down to skull bones, 209
    examination of, 111–13
    Frankfurt plane and, 220–21, 223
    severed, difficult to examine, 209
    severed, eeriness of, 208
    weight of, 208–9
head injuries, 112–13
headless corpses, 264–65
heart, 95, 103, 104, 105
    blood circulation and, 39, 40, 70, 73,
        107
    removal and examination of, 106,
        107–8
heart attacks, 106, 107, 171, 263
heart disease, 110
height, 24
Helpern, Milton, 262–63
Hemings, Sally, 145, 187
heroin, 215
    in Binion case, 63, 68, 69, 72, 73, 75,
        84–85, 87–90
    chasing the dragon and, 68, 75, 85
hiatal hernia, 105
high blood pressure, 109
Hitler, Adolf, 182
HIV, 96
Hoadley, R. Bruce, 125–26
Hoffa, Jimmy, 61, 62
Holmes, Sherlock, 126–27
homicide, 75, 100, 110, 138
    change in nature of, 143–44
homicide autopsies, 15–32, 102–18
    clear thinking in, 17–18
    collecting samples in, 27–30
    detectives' briefings in, 24–26
    examination of wounds in, 30
    extreme measures in, 113–15
    fainting during, 17
    fingerprinting in, 26
    information requested from crime
        scene during, 16–17, 29, 113
    medical examiner's independence and
        neutrality in, 15
    people present during, 15, 111–12
    photographing body in, 24, 28–29
    removing bags from hands in, 26
    removing body from bag in, 20
    removing clothes from body in, 29

search of body bag in, 20
specimens saved as evidence in, 117
in strangulation case, 24–32, 102–18
tag on body and, 21–22
tattoos examined in, 30–32
unzipping of body bag in, 17, 18
visual inspection in, 26–27, 30–32
X rays in, 29–30, 195
Hoover, J. Edgar, 127
hospitals, deaths in, 22, 98
Howell, Linda, 162–63

Iannarelli, Alfred, 224
identification:
    dental evidence and, 113, 114, 115,
        125, 183, 192, 207, 210, 212–15,
        264–65
    DNA and, 144–46, 184–85, 207,
        212
    ear prints and, 224
    of exhumed remains, 180, 182–85,
        192, 265–66
    facial reconstruction and, 209,
        220–24
    of loved one's body, 23, 222
    misidentification and, 22–23
    natural decay halted for, 207
    rebuilding with fragments and,
        207–8
    of Romanovs' remains, 180, 182–85,
        214, 265–66
    of skeletonized bodies, 211–12
    tags and, 21–22
    in TWA Flight 800 crash, 61–62
incisions, 95–97, 111
insect bites, 169, 171
insect nets, 166, 167
insects, 158–75, 209, 256–57, 260–61
    auto accidents and, 163, 171
    charred and burned flesh and,
        161–62, 256
    collecting samples of, 166–67
    courtroom testimony on, 165–66,
        168
    eggs of, 167
    identifying species of, 170–71
    place of death and, 169
    sex of, 171
    specimen preservation and, 167,
        168–69
    succession of, 170, 173
    temperature data and, 163–64,
        167–68, 171
    time of death and, 162–64, 166–73
    various information discerned from,
        171–72

Index

Institute on the Physical Significance of
    Human Bloodstain Evidence,
    36–56
insurance, 66–67, 171, 213
Internet, 91–92
intravenous lines and tubes, 22

Jack the Ripper, 28–29, 140
James, Jesse, 187
jaws, 113, 150
Jefferson, Thomas, 145, 187
Jeffreys, Alec, 144
jewelry, 27
John, King of England, 99–100
joint tattoos, 31
judges:
    admissibility of evidence and, 80–82
    juries instructed on expert witnesses
      by, 82, 84
    qualifying process and, 80, 81,
      165–66, 234, 243
junk science, 229–49
    credentialing process and, 243–45
    in death penalty cases, 234, 237, 239,
      241–43
    defined, 233
    of Erdmann, 239–41
    motivations for, 231–33
    nonscientific evidence contaminated
      by, 237
    phrenology as, 233–34
    predicting future behavior of con-
      victed as, 242–43
    technology and, 245–47
    of Zain, 229–31, 235–39, 241, 248
juries, 60, 81, 92
    in capital cases in Texas, 242
    DNA results and, 145–46
    exhumations and, 196
    expert witnesses and, 77, 82, 84, 86
    forensic animation software and,
      245–47
    insurance claims and, 66, 67
Justice Department, U.S., 247

Kaddish, 181
Kardashian, Robert, 146
Kennedy, Edward, 189
Kennedy, John F., 20, 24, 91, 99,
    100–101, 116
Kennedy, Robert F., 37
kidneys, 103, 109
King, Martin Luther, Jr., 37, 91, 98, 99,
    193

Kish, Paul Erwin, 37, 53–55
Kopechne, Mary Jo, 189
Kosovo, 190
Ku Klux Klan, 199, 202
Kunstler, William, 140–42

land mines, 261
Langmuir, Irving, 232
LAPD, 26, 146–53
    see also Simpson case
Lauridson, James, 201
Lavater, Johann Caspar, 224
lay experts, 80
Lee, Henry C., 121–34, 146–48, 197,
    259, 261, 267
    background of, 127, 128–29
    model crime lab built by, 129–31
    talks given by, 127–28, 132–33
    wood chipper case and, 123–26
Lee, Margaret Song, 128–29
legs, 113
Lenin, V. I., 181, 182, 183
Lennon, John, 116
Levine, Lowell, 114, 125, 180, 183, 193,
    213–14, 266
Lewinsky, Monica, 132
Lewis, Meriwether, 187
lice, 171, 172, 265
lifestyle:
    facial reconstruction and, 221, 223
    reflected in death, 19, 104, 105
ligature, 24–25, 27
light, searching for semen with, 26, 30
Lincoln, Abraham, 188
lint, 26
liposuction, 265
lip prints, 210, 224
lips, 208
Litman, Jack, 131
liver, 103, 105, 109
livor mortis (lividity), 19, 20, 32, 40, 47,
    150
Locard, Edmund, 127
Locard's Exchange Principle, 21
Lord, Wayne, 173, 265
"Love Bug" case, 263–64
Luce, Clare Boothe, 220
lungs, 104, 105
    removal and examination of, 108–9

MacDonell, Herbert Leon, 36–56, 81
    Mowbray case and, 50–53
    résumé of, 37–38
    Simpson case and, 45–48

Index

MacDonell, Phyllis, 44, 53
maggots, *see* insects
MAGNA™ Brush, 38
manner of death, 16, 59–61, 75, 201–2
  incorrect assumptions about, 62–64, 67–79
  never determined, 60–61
manuscripts, exhumation of, 185–86
Maples, William, 183
Marlowe, Christopher, 186
masks, for autopsies, 18
mass graves, 190
mastoiditis, 24
masturbation, 263
medical examiners, 100–101, 234–35
  assistant, author's first job as, 138–40
  contemporaneous notes of, 26, 74, 116–17
  documents generated by, 117; *see also* autopsy reports
  independence and neutrality of, 15, 73–74
  payment of, 83
  reporting of death to, 97–98
  respect for dead required of, 97, 101–2, 115
  reviewing work of, 74
  in Simpson case, 150–52
medical history, 140, 192
Mengele, Joseph, 214
menstruation, 110
microsatellites, 144
misidentifications, 22–23
missing people, 60–61, 62
mites, 173
mitochondrial DNA, 184, 210, 212
Momot, John, 72
Montand, Yves, 188
morgues, 14–15, 22, 91, 138
  eating in, 26
  insect evidence in, 168
  live bodies in, 23
  see also autopsies; homicide autopsies
mosquitoes, 171, 172
mouth, 221
  blood spraying out of, 53–56
  see also jaw; teeth and dental work
moving body after death:
  by police, 46–47, 152
  signs of, 32, 169
Mowbray, Susie and William, 50–53
mucus, 145
Murphy, Sandy, 63–64, 68, 69, 72–73, 85–92

muscles, facial, 222
My Cousin Vinny, 80, 82

Napoleon Bonaparte, 218–20
Native Americans, 212, 254–55, 267
natural death, 75, 207
neck, 210
  examination of, 110–11
necrophilia, 260
neglect, 169
Newsweek, 165
Newton, Wayne, 253, 254–55, 267
New York Post, 116
Nicholas II, Tsar, 179, 180, 181–85, 266
Nikitin, Sergei Alekseevich, 265–66
nose, 210, 221
notes, of autopsy, 26, 74, 116–17
notices of death, 117
Novum Organum (Bacon), 231
nuclear (genomic) DNA, 184, 197, 210

Oakes, Cathryn, 183
O'Block, Robert, 244–45
occipital bone, 210
"Oddball Case," 261–62
opinion testimony, 82–83
organs, examination of, 103, 105–13
Oswald, Lee Harvey, 24

panniculus, 103
Parkman, George, 212–13
paternity, establishing of, 145, 186–88
pathological science, 232, 241
pathology, 80
  see also forensic pathology
Paul, Henri, 215–18
Pauling, Linus, 232
penicillin, 97, 108
pericardial sac, 106
perimeter, at crime scene, 148–49
petechial hemorrhage, 70–71, 74, 76, 77
Peters, Ed, 193
Philip, Prince of England, 184, 185
photographs, 224
  in autopsies, 24, 28–29, 115–16
  of crime scenes, 28–29, 46, 48, 152, 263
  on driver's licenses, 23
phrenology, 233–34
physicians, as expert witnesses, 89
place of death, signs of moved body and, 32, 169
plasma, 40
plea bargaining, 69, 153

Index

PMS, 110
Pocahontas, 254–55, 267
poisons, 190, 219–20
police, 153
  at autopsies, 15, 16, 60, 111–12
  at crime scenes, 26, 46–48, 59, 63, 64, 148–53, 263
  evidence disrupted by, 26, 46–48, 63, 148–53
  see also detectives
polygraphs, 82
polymorphisms, 144
preliminary hearings, 70, 82
  in Binion case, 70, 76, 78, 84–88, 89
"Preppy Murderer," 131
presidents, exhumation of, 187–88
proof:
  burden of, 153
  degrees of, 84
prosecution, 60, 233
  burden of proof on, 153
  compelled to reveal evidence to defense, 77, 108
  evidence concealed or falsified by, 247
  job of, 78
Pruitt, Vann, 199–200, 202
public defenders, 248

qualifying process, 79–82, 234, 243
  credentialing business and, 243–45
  forensic entomology and, 165–66

race, 211, 212, 216, 221
radar, ground penetrating (GPR), 190–91
Ramsey, JonBenet, 63, 101, 148
rape, 132–33, 144, 172, 247
  Zain's junk science and, 229–31
rape kits, 27–30, 145, 152
rebreather devices, 18, 19
red blood cells, 40, 72, 103, 197
Redi, Francesco, 159
Rembrandt, 26
Reno, forensic science convention in, 253–67
respect for human body, 97, 101–2, 115–16, 209
Ressler, Robert, 264
Revere, Paul, 212
rheumatic fever, 108
rib cage, cutting through, 104
Richard I, King of England, 99
rigor mortis, 19, 20, 150
Rodriguez, Bill, 201
Rogers, David, 69, 76–78, 85

Rokitansky procedure, 106
Romanov family, 91, 180, 181–85
  execution of, 181–82
  identification of remains of, 180, 182–85, 214, 265–66
Rosner, Richard, 257
Rossetti, Dante Gabriel, 185–86
Rupp, Joe, 263–64
Ryabov, Gely, 181, 182–83

Sacco case, 114
saliva, 26, 29, 145
Salter, Sarah Edwards, 201, 202
Sanctity of the Sepulchre, 102, 189
scalpels, 95–96, 102
scalp incisions, 111
scenes of death, 138–40
  see also crime scenes
Schanzkowska, Franzisca, 185
science, 231–32
  bad, *see* junk science
  see also forensic science; *specific fields*
Scotland Yard, 127
screwworms, 163
scrubs, 18
semen, 145, 263
  searching for traces of, 26, 30
serial killers, 214, 264, 265
sex, 25, 26, 27, 30, 65, 108
  autoerotic deaths and, 263–64
shag rugs, evidence concealed in, 142–43
Shakespeare, William, 186
Shapiro, Bob, 142–43, 146–47
sheets, wrapping bodies in, 20
Shellow, Jim, 90, 91
Sheppard, Sam and Marilyn, 37, 246
shrouds, 13
sickle-cell anemia, 109
Siddal, Elizabeth, 185–86
Simms, Larry, 68–71, 73–79, 84–85, 90
Simpson, Nicole Brown, 45–48, 64, 92, 146, 150
  failure to collect blood drops on back of, 46–47, 152
  mishandling of body of, 46–48, 150–52
  see also Simpson case
Simpson, O.J., 64
  author's connections to, 140–43
  author's examination of, 115, 146–47
Simpson case, 32, 37, 45–48, 67, 91, 92, 146–53, 164
  assumption of quick confession in, 64
  DNA testimony in, 87
  failure to protect crime scene in, 26, 140, 148–53

Lee's involvement in, 131, 134
medical examiner's late arrival in, 150–52
sloppy photographic work in, 152
situs inversus, 105
skeletonized bodies, 210, 211–12
sketches (two-dimensional reconstructions), 222–24
skin, 104, 115, 145, 208, 210, 221
skull, 112, 208, 209, 211
    facial reconstruction and, 113, 209, 220–24, 266
slaves, 187, 188
slippage, 27
smell:
    in autopsies, 17, 18–19, 27
    of death, insects and, 159, 171
Smith, William Kennedy, 131
smoking, 105, 108, 221
software, forensic animation, 245–47
soil samples, exhumation and, 190
specialties, medical, 80
sperm, 26, 27, 30, 184
spleen, 109
Starrs, Jim, 186–87, 197
starry sky effect, 195
sternum, 104
stomach, 16, 105, 106
    removal and examination of, 109
stranger murders, 143
strangulation, 71, 96
    autopsy in case of, 24–32, 102–18
    erection and, 28
suffocation, 71, 76, 88, 90, 240
    burking and, 76–77, 85
suicide, 19, 52, 75, 89–90, 99, 100, 105, 110, 139
    family's response to, 65, 66
    incorrect assumptions and, 63–64, 65
    insurance claims and, 66–67
    presumption against, in courts, 65–67
Sullivan, Mary, 196–98
sun exposure, 221
Sung Tz'u, 159
Supreme Court, U.S., 81, 234, 241, 242
surface tension, 40–41
suspect profiling, 144
sutures, in cranium, 210
swabs, 27, 30
swallowing enough of anything to cause death, 75
syphilis, 108

Tabish, Rick, 68, 69, 85–92
tags, on bodies, 21–22, 28

tape recorders, for autopsy notes, 26
tattoos, 30–32
taxes, on unnatural deaths, 99–100
Taylor, Zachary, 188
technology, junk science and, 245–47
teeth and dental work, 221
    identifications made from, 113, 114, 115, 125, 183, 192, 207, 210, 212–15, 264–65
television, 91, 200
temperature:
    body, after death, 19–20, 150
    insects and, 163–64, 167–68, 171
Teriipia, Tarita, 141, 142
testes, 105, 110, 262
Texas:
    attempts to predict future violence of convicted in, 242–43
    death penalty cases in, 241–43, 248–49
    Zain's and Erdmann's junk science in, 235, 238, 239–41
Thin Blue Line, The, 242
time of death, 107
    body changes after death and, 19–20, 32
    bruises and, 72
    evidence at scene and, 16
    insects and, 162–64, 166–73
    in Simpson case, 150, 151
Tinning, Mary Beth, 99
tissue samples, 71
Tomb of the Unknowns, 188–89
tongue, 210
tongue test, 211
toxicology, 106
trace evidence:
    collected in autopsies, 27–30
    at crime scene, protecting and collecting of, 21, 29, 63, 64, 145–46, 148–53
    DNA and, 144–46
    in illicit burials, 190
trade shows, 258–59
trials, *see* court proceedings; judges; juries; preliminary hearings
Trosper, Terri, 239–40
TWA Flight 800, 61–62, 214
two-dimensional reconstructions, 222–24
Tylenol, 19

undetermined cause or manner of death, 60–61, 75
Union of Concerned Scientists, 233

Index

unknown soldier, exhumation of, 188–89
unnatural deaths, 207
    autopsies in, 98–99
    lack of uniform method for examina-
        tion of, 100–101
    tax in medieval England on, 99–100
urine samples, 106
uterus, 110

Vannatter, Philip, 149
Venus (slave), 187
vertebrae, 210
Victoria, Queen of England, 184
Virchow method, 106
von Bulow, Claus, 37, 91

Wall, David, 69, 76–78, 91
wallpaper, arsenic in, 219–20
Walsingham, Sir Thomas, 186
Warren, Joseph, 212
Washing Away of Wrongs, The (Sung), 159
Washington, George, 186, 187
Washington, John Augustine, 187
wasps, 172–73
Webster, John White, 212–13
Wecht, Cyril, 89–90, 91
weight, 24
West Virginia, Zain's junk science in,
    229–31, 235–38, 239, 248

West Virginia Supreme Court, 231,
    237–38, 239
Wetli, Charles, 61
white blood cells, 40, 72, 197
wintergreen oil, 18, 27
wishful science, 231–32
witnesses, 133, 146
    see also expert witnesses
women, 110, 211
    in autopsies, 17
Woodall, Glen, 230–31
wood analysis, 125–26
"Wood Chipper Murder," 123–26
Woods Light, 26, 30
wounds:
    examination of, 30
    gunshot, 51
wrongful arrests, 247
wrongful convictions:
    DNA in overturning of, 230–31, 237,
        238, 247
    junk science and, 229–31, 235–39

Xanax, in Binion case, 63, 68–69,
    73–76, 84–85, 87, 89
X rays, 29–30, 193, 195, 213

Y incision, 95–97, 111

Zain, Fred, 229–31, 235–39, 241, 248